Aids to Ophthalmology

To our wives

Aids to Ophthalmology

P. T. Khaw *
MRCP FRCS DO
Senior Registrar in Ophthalmology
Moorfields Eye Hospital, London

D. S. Hughes *
FRCS DO
Ophthalmologist
Bawku Hospital, Burkina Faso

S. J. Keightley *
BSc FRCS DO
Consultant Ophthalmologist
Basingstoke District Hospital

R. F. Walters *
BSc FRCS DO
Senior Registrar in Ophthalmology
Queen Alexandra Hospital, Portsmouth

A. R. Elkington
MA FRCS DO
Senior Lecturer/Consultant Ophthalmologist
University of Southampton/Southampton Eye Hospital

*formerly of Southampton Eye Hospital

CHURCHILL LIVINGSTONE
EDINBURGH LONDON MELBOURNE AND NEW YORK 1989

CHURCHILL LIVINGSTONE
Medical Division of Longman Group UK Limited

Distributed in the United States of America by
Churchill Livingstone Inc., 1560 Broadway, New
York, N.Y. 10036, and by associated companies,
branches and representatives throughout the
world.

First Edition 1989

ISBN 0-443-04012-5

British Library Cataloguing in Publication Data
Aids to ophthalmology.
1. Ophthalmology
I. Khaw, P. T. II. Series
617.7

Library of Congress Cataloging in Publication Data
Aids to ophthalmology / P. T. Khaw . . . [et al.]. —
1st ed.
    p. cm.
  Bibliography: p.
  Includes index.
    1. Ophthalmology — Handbooks, manuals,
etc. 2. Eye — Diseases — Handbooks, manuals,
etc.   I. Khaw, P. T. (Peng T.)
  [DNLM: 1. Eye Diseases. 2. Ophthalmology.
WW 100 A288]
RE48.9.A33 1989
617.7 — dc19
DNLM/DLC
for Library of Congress   88-36959
                                               CIP

Produced by Longman Singapore Publishers (Pte) Ltd.
Printed in Singapore

Preface

This book is intended primarily as a revision text for those sitting examinations for either a Diploma in Ophthalmology or a Fellowship of one of the Royal Colleges. We have tried to strike a balance between basic science and clinical ophthalmology, particularly in view of the forthcoming 'modular' format of these examinations. It is also our hope that advanced medical students, optometrists and ophthalmic nurses will find this book useful.

Our aim has been to provide a basic, pocket-sized text to which readers can add to create a personal aide-memoire. By its very nature it cannot be considered to be fully comprehensive but it may help readers to identify gaps in their knowledge and stimulate further reading.

1989

P. T. K.
D. S. H.
S. J. K.
R. F. W.
A. R. E.

Acknowledgements

We thank our colleagues who have helped us with their advice and criticism. We extend our warm appreciation to Peggy Khaw and Anna Quick for their patience and for the many hours they spent working on the manuscript. The help that Sarah Lawrence and Peggy Robinson gave us over the references was invaluable. Finally, we express our appreciation to Peter Jack who drew the diagrams.

Contents

Contents

Eyelids

EYELID MARGINS

1. Palpebral aperture — 30 mm long × 10 mm high
2. Eyelid margins — divided into lateral $\frac{5}{6}$ and medial $\frac{1}{6}$ by lacrimal puncta
   a. Lateral margin — 2 mm thick, rounded anterior edge, perpendicular/posterior edge
      (i) Anteriorly
         Lashes. 2–3 rows. Longer in upper lid and in children. Curved away from opposite lid. No erector muscles. 10 week growth, 5 months resting phase
         Glands of Moll. Modified sweat glands, 2 mm long
         Glands of Zeis. Sebaceous glands, 2 per lash
      (ii) Posteriorly
         Meibomian gland openings. 25 upper lid, 20 lower lid
         Grey line. Vascular watershed. Splits easily with minimal bleeding. Junction of anterior and posterior lamellae
   b. Medial margin — both edges rounded, no lashes or glands. Forms boundaries of lacus lacrimalis

ANTERIOR LAMELLA OF LID

1. Skin — fine texture, thin and elastic. Attached to deep fascia at medial and lateral canthus and at orbital margins. No subcutaneous fat
2. Orbicularis muscle
   a. Three portions:
      (i) Orbital. Origin — medial palpebral ligament and adjacent bone. Sweeps round lateral canthus
      (ii) Palpebral. Origin — medial palpebral ligament. Sweeps across upper and lower tarsal plates (pretarsal) and orbital septum (preseptal). Interdigitates to form lateral palpebral raphé
      (iii) Lacrimal (Horner's muscle). Origin — posterior lacrimal crest. Fibres pass along the canaliculi to the tarsal plates extending to the lateral palpebral raphé

1

b. Nerve supply. Upper branches of 7th entering deeply
c. Function.
   (i) Orbital — forcible closure of lids
   (ii) Palpebral — blinking
   (iii) Lacrimal — tear drainage

POSTERIOR LAMELLA OF LID

1. Tarsal plate — fibrous, scaphoid-shaped skeleton of lid in which Meibomian glands are embedded. 30 mm long × 10 mm (upper). 30 mm long × 5 mm (lower). Stretches between palpebral ligaments and continuous with orbital septum. Meibomian glands — 10–15 acini round central duct producing oily secretion
2. Conjunctiva

ORBITAL SEPTUM

1. Extension of periorbita from orbital rim to tarsal plates
2. Weaker inferiorly and medial upper lid
3. Pierced by levator palpebrae superioris, lower lid retractor, nerves and vessels

LEVATOR PALPEBRAE SUPERIORIS

1. Origin — lesser wing of sphenoid
2. Insertion
   a. Skin of lid (palpebral furrow)
   b. Medial and lateral palpebral ligament
   c. Anterior surface of tarsal plate
   d. Pre-tarsal orbicularis
3. Relations
   a. Lies above superior rectus
   b. Separated from orbital roof by 4th and frontal nerves (5a)
   c. Approximately 40 mm long, ending 10 mm behind orbital septum in an aponeurosis
   d. Condensation running from trochlea to lacrimal gland (Whitnall's ligament)
   e. Passes through septum 4 mm above tarsus
4. Function
   a. Raises upper lid (approximately 10 mm)
   b. Acts in synergism with superior rectus
5. Nerve supply — 3rd nerve (upper division) entering deep surface

MÜLLER'S MUSCLE

1. Origin — aponeurosis of levator palpebrae superioris
2. Insertion — Upper edge of tarsus
3. Function — raises upper lid (approximately 2 mm)
4. Nerve supply — sympathetic via superior cervical ganglion

INFERIOR RETRACTOR

1. Forward extension of fascia from inferior rectus
2. Surrounds inferior oblique as Lockwood's ligament
3. Inserts into
   a. Lower fornix
   b. Lower edge of tarsus
   c. Anterior surface of tarsus
4. Has smooth muscle component which lowers lower lid 1 mm

PALPEBRAL LIGAMENTS

1. Medial — 4 mm long and 2 mm wide
   Palpable, overlying inferior portion of lacrimal sac
   Angular vein lies superficially
2. Lateral — 7 mm long and 2 mm wide
   Separated from lateral palpebral raphé by palpebral
   portion of lacrimal gland

BLOOD SUPPLY TO EYELIDS

1. Arterial
   a. Marginal arcade 3–4 mm from lid margin
   b. Deep peripheral arcade (upper lid only)
   c. Supplied by medial palpebral arteries and lateral palpebral
      arteries. Anastomosis between extracranial and intracranial
      supply
2. Venous
   Watershed area, connection between intracranial and
   extracranial drainage

LYMPHATIC DRAINAGE OF EYELIDS

1. Submandibular nodes — drain medial $\frac{1}{3}$ of upper lid; medial $\frac{2}{3}$
   of lower lid
2. Preauricular nodes — drain lateral $\frac{2}{3}$ of upper lid; lateral $\frac{1}{3}$ of
   lower lid

SENSORY NERVE SUPPLY TO EYELIDS

1. Upper lid — ophthalmic division of 5th (5a)
2. Lower lid — maxillary division of 5th (5b)

FUNCTION OF LIDS

1. Protection of eye
2. Reconstitution of tear film
3. Coverage of eye during sleep

REQUIREMENTS FOR NORMAL LID FUNCTION

1. Normal lid height
2. Normal lid movement
3. Normal muscle tone
4. Normal blinking and reflex movement
5. Normal lid contour

BLINKING

1. Reflex
   a. Sensory stimuli. Latency 100 ms. Persists in decerebrate state
   b. Optical stimuli. Slower reflex due to central connections. Absent in children. 2 aspects: (i) dazzle (subcortical); (ii) menace (cortical)
2. Voluntary
3. Spontaneous
   a. Involuntary
   b. Rate — 12/min set by globus pallidus. Reduced by alcohol. Increased by emotion
   c. Amplitude — 9.5 mm
   d. Duration — 330 ms
   e. Total occlusion time — 150 ms

EMBRYOLOGY

1. Eyelid folds form at 8 weeks of gestation
2. Upper lid formed by fusion of medial and lateral frontonasal processes
3. Lower lid formed by fusion of lateral maxillary processes and medial nasal processes
4. Lid folds meet and fuse at 12 weeks, separating from nasal side at 24 weeks. Plica forms at the same time

CONGENITAL ABNORMALITIES

1. Ankyloblepharon — adhesion between lids
2. Ablepharon — absence of lids
3. Coloboma — notching of upper lid. Associated with epidermoid cysts
4. Distichiasis — extra row of lashes from Meibomian orifices

directed backwards. Treatment — lid split and posterior lamellar cryotherapy
5. Epicanthus — medial skin fold obscuring caruncle. The most common congenital variation, especially in Mongoloid races. A common cause of pseudoesotropia
6. Ptosis
   a. Simple. Unilateral. Dystrophy of levator palpebrae superioris with or without reduced superior rectus function. Features
      (i) Absent skin crease
      (ii) Frontalis overaction
      (iii) Chin up head position
      (iv) Amblyopia if ptosis causes occlusion
      Surgery at 4 years if uncomplicated
   b. Jaw Winking. Unilateral. Associated with paradoxical elevation on lateral jaw movement. Improves with age
   c. Blepharophimosis. Autosomal dominant. Bilateral ptosis with inverted epicanthus, ectropion and wide intercanthal distance
7. Ectropion — rare
8. Entropion
   a. Bilateral, mild, affecting lower lid
   b. Especially in Mongoloid races
   c. Hypertrophy of skin and orbicularis
   d. Self limiting by 2 years
   e. Treatment — excision of strip of skin and orbicularis

ACQUIRED DISORDERS

Entropion
1. Involutional
   a. Affects lower lid
   b. Pathology
      (i) Preseptal overriding pretarsal orbicularis
      (ii) Horizontal lid laxity due to stretched canthal tendons and orbital fat atrophy
      (iii) Weakened tarsus allowing flexure
      (iv) Vertical instability due to dehiscence of retractors
   c. Treatment
      (i) Taping of lid or eversion sutures if unfit
      (ii) Surgical correction of any or all above features, e.g. Wies' or Wheeler's operations
2. Cicatricial
   a. Affects upper or lower lid
   b. Pathology — scarring and shortening of posterior lamella
   c. Causes
      (i) Trachoma
      (ii) Stevens-Johnson syndrome

       (iii) Radiation
       (iv) Chemical injury
       (v) Surgery
       (vi) Lacerations
       (vii) Benign mucous membrane pemphigoid
    d. Treatment of upper lid entropion
       (i) Minimal: anterior lamellar reposition with or without lash removal
       (ii) Moderate: as for minimal + tarsal wedge resection
       (iii) Severe: tarsal split, 180° rotation or posterior lamellar graft
3. Acute spastic
    a. Pathology — spasm of orbicularis with ocular irritation or essential blepharospasm. Associated with involutional entropion
    b. Treatment
       (i) Removal of irritation
       (ii) Treatment of associated involutional entropion
       (iii) Injection of botulinum toxin into orbicularis
       (iv) Partial 7th nerve section

Ectropion
1. Involutional
    a. Usually lower lid
    b. Pathology
       (i) Horizontal lid laxity related to canthal tendon stretching
       (ii) Pretarsal orbicularis weakness
    c. Treatment
       (i) Cicatrization by cautery
       (ii) Conjunctivoplasty
       (iii) Horizontal lid shortening
2. Cicatricial
    a. Upper or lower lid
    b. Causes
       (i) Trauma: lacerations, burns, surgery
       (ii) Tumours
       (iii) Infections
    c. Treatment
       (i) Prevention of exposure
       (ii) Release of scarring, e.g. Z-plasty, skin grafting
3. Paralytic
    a. Lower lid
    b. Causes muscular or 7th nerve disorders
    c. Treatment
       (i) Prevention of exposure and corneal drying
       (ii) Tarsorrhaphy
       (iii) Circlage, lid weights and magnets
       (iv) Nerve transposition or graft

Ptosis
1. Neurogenic
   a. 3rd nerve palsy
   b. Horner's syndrome
   c. Jaw winking
   d. Aberrant 3rd nerve regeneration
2. Myogenic
   a. Congenital
   b. Acquired
      (i) Myasthenia gravis — abnormality of neuromuscular junction. Variable fatiguable ptosis. Cogan's twitch sign
      (ii) Dystrophia myotonica — autosomal dominant. Bilateral ptosis with frontalis overaction
      (iii) Mitochondrial myopathy — bilateral ptosis with ophthalmoplegia
3. Aponeurotic
   a. Dehiscence of levator palpebrae superioris aponeurosis
   b. Causes
      (i) Senility
      (ii) Trauma
4. Mechanical
   Causes
   a. Tumours, e.g. chalazion
   b. Inflammation, e.g. vernal catarrh
   c. Oedema, e.g. dermatochalasis
   d. Conjunctival scarring
   e. Trauma, e.g Postoperative

Assessment of ptosis
1. Exclude pseudoptosis, e.g. microphthalmos, cornea plana, or hypertropia in eye with 'ptosis' or lid retraction, prominent eye, hypotropia in other eye
2. Measure levator function (immobilize frontalis). Normal: 15 mm or greater
3. Measure degree of ptosis
4. Check ocular motility
5. Ask patient to move jaw (jaw-winking)
6. Check Bell's phenomenon
7. Assess corneal sensation
8. Assess tear film and secretion
9. General examination
10. Consider Tensilon test

Treatment of ptosis
1. Treat underlying condition, e.g. anticholinesterases in myasthenia gravis
2. Spectacle props (ptosis crutches), haptic contact lenses
3. Lubricate as there is a higher risk of corneal exposure,

especially with myogenic causes of ptosis
4. Surgery — proportional to
   a. levator function
   b. degree of ptosis

Bacterial infections and inflammations of the eyelids
1. Stye — infected gland of Zeis
2. Chalazion — chronic inflammation of a Meibomian gland
   associated with blepharitis
   a. Histopathology — lipogranuloma with foreign body giant
      cells, fibrosis, and fluid content
   b. Treatment
      (i) Conservative — hot compresses and topical antibiotics
      (ii) Surgery — incision and curettage
3. Meibomianitis — passive retention of inspissated secretions
4. Blepharitis
   a. Inflammation of the lid margin
   b. Types
      (i) Staphylococcal (*Staph aureus, Staph epidermidis*)
      (ii) Seborrhoeic (*Diphtheroids, Pityrosporum ovale*)
   c. Symptoms — ocular irritation
   d. Signs — Staphylococcal
      (i) Trichiasis
      (ii) Madarosis
      (iii) Poliosis
      (iv) Marginal keratitis
      (v) Papillary conjunctivitis
          — Seborrhoeic
      (i) Greasy scales
      (ii) Chalazia
      (iii) Punctate epithelial erosions
   e. Treatment
      (i) Lid hygiene
      (ii) Lubricants
      (iii) Topical antibiotics
      (iv) Systemic antibiotics, e.g. oxytetracycline
5. Occasional infections
   a. Impetigo
   b. Erysipelas
   c. Anthrax
   d. Tuberculosis
   e. Syphilis
6. Granuloma pyogenicum — granulation tissue related to
   bacterial infection

Viral infections
1. Herpes simplex
2. Herpes zoster

3. Viral warts
   a. Filiform lesions
   b. Histopathology — parakeratosis, vacuolated nuclei with eosinophilic inclusions
4. Molluscum contagiosum
   a. 'Water warts' — umbilicated contagious lesions associated with a follicular conjunctivitis
   b. Histopathology — distended epithelial cells containing eosinophilic bodies which stain with Lugol's iodine
   c. Treatment — expression and chemical cautery

Fungal infections and infestations
1. Tinea infections (ringworm)
2. Lice
3. Myiasis (fly maggots)
4. Onchocerciasis

Trichiasis
Backwardly directed lashes causing irritation. Related to scarring of the eyelids
1. Causes
   a. Staphylococcal blepharitis
   b. Past herpes zoster ophthalmicus
   c. Trauma (physical, chemical and irradiation)
   d. Conjunctival scarring diseases
2. Treatment
   a. Epilation
   b. Soft contact lens
   c. Cryotherapy
   d. Electrolysis

Lagophthalmos
Inadequate eyelid closure
1. Associations
   a. Race (Mongoloid)
   b. Nocturnal
   c. 7th nerve palsy
   d. Proptosis
   e. Lid retraction
   f. Buphthalmos
2. Treatment
   a. Lubricants
   b. Lid taping
   c. Tarsorrhaphy

Causes of reduced blinking
1. Progressive supranuclear palsy
2. Parkinson's disease

3. Hyperthyroidism
4. Reduced conscious level
5. Drugs, e.g. alcohol

Blepharoclonus
1. Exaggerated reflex blinking with increased frequency and contraction
2. Associations
   a. Ocular irritation
   b. Tic

Orbicularis Myokymia
1. Involuntary contraction giving an annoying twitching sensation
2. Related to fatigue and occasionally hemifacial spasm and multiple sclerosis

Blepharospasm
1. Involuntary tonic, spasmodic, bilateral eyelid closure. Usually occurs over the age of 60 years
2. Causes
   a. Idiopathic
   b. Parkinson's disease
   c. Psychogenic
   d. Postencephalitic
   e. Tetany

Causes of lid swelling
1. Local causes, e.g. allergy, infection
2. Dysthyroid states
3. Nephrotic syndrome
4. Angioneurotic oedema
5. Premenstrual syndrome
6. Infiltrates, e.g. myeloma

Xanthelasma
Fatty plaque at medial end of the eyelids (usually bilateral)
1. Associations
   a. Primary hyperlipidaemic states
   b. Diabetes mellitus
   c. Hypothyroidism
   d. Primary biliary cirrhosis
   e. Histiocytosis X
2. Histopathology — foam cells (macrophages) in epidermis
3. Management
   a. Exclude underlying cause
   b. Excision (60% recurrence)

Benign tumours
1. Basal cell papilloma (seborrhoeic keratosis)
   a. Common, sessile
   b. Histopathology — basal cell proliferation with keratin nests
2. Squamous cell papilloma
   a. Common, sessile or pedunculated
   b. Histopathology — excessive convoluted epithelium. Central fibrovascular core. Keratin horn formation
3. Solar Keratosis
   a. Flat, multiple, scaly lesions. Occasionally papillomatous with horn formation. Premalignant
   b. Histopathology — Dysplastic epithelium with pronounced keratosis. No invasion
4. Keratoacanthoma
   a. Enlarges over months, then regresses. Volcano-shaped with keratin plug
   b. Histopathology — difficult to differentiate from squamous cell carcinoma unless whole lesion examined histologically. Hyperplastic epithelium. Parakeratosis, hyperkeratosis. No invasion but basal inflammation
5. Haemangioma
   a. Strawberry naevus. Evident in neonatal period. Grows then usually regresses by 5 years of age
   b. Histopathology — proliferation of capillaries, some of which are not canalized
6. Neurofibroma
   a. Associated with neurofibromatosis
   b. Histopathology — Nodular proliferation of Schwann's cells and fibroblasts. Staining for S100 protein shows neuroectodermal origin
7. Naevi
   a. Congenital collections of naevus cells. Pigmented or nonpigmented. May develop pigmentation after puberty
   b. Histopathology — naevus cells stain uniformly blue with H & E. Classified according to location within skin
      (i) Epidermal — slightly thickened epithelium with naevus cells forming cysts
      (ii) Junctional — activity at epidermal/dermal junction, occuring in children or at puberty
      (iii) Dermal — fascicles of naevus cells within the dermis. Diffuse dermal naevus or naevus of Ota associated with choroidal melanomas
      (iv) Compound — malignant

Malignant tumours
1. Basal cell carcinoma
   a. Most common malignant tumour of the eyelids
   b. Medial lower lid commonest site

   c. Do not metastasize
   d. Types
      (i) Nodulo-ulcerative. Well defined
         Histopathology — palisaded basal cell proliferation with
         invasion and cyst formation. Ulceration and
         inflammation
      (ii) Sclerosing (morphoea)
         Histopathology — islands of basal cells infiltrating
         beneath epidermis. Multifocal. Can also be divided into
         solid, cystic, adenoid, keratotic and fibrosing types
         histologically
   e. Treatment
      (i) Cryotherapy — 10% recurrence rate
      (ii) Radiotherapy — not for inner canthal area
     (iii) Surgical — recurrence in only 25% of those with
         histologically incomplete excision
2. Squamous cell carcinoma
   a. Arise de novo
   b. Arise from premalignant states such as solar keratoses,
      arsenical keratoses and xeroderma pigmentosum
   c. May metastasize to lymph nodes
   d. Histopathology — depends on degree of differentiation
      ranging from well-differentiated keratinizing carcinomas
      (with cell nests and keratin pearls) to anaplastic spindle cell
      growths. May evoke a chronic inflammatory response
3. Carcinoma-in-situ (Bowen's disease)
   a. Upper lid most common site
   b. 5% of eyelid tumours
   c. Everted edges
   d. Histopathology — dedifferentiation of epithelial cells.
      Changes are localized to epidermis. Transition to squamous
      cell carcinoma may occur
4. Meibomian gland carcinoma
   a. Rare
   b. Localized. May present as recurrent chalazion
   c. Diffuse. May present as persistent chronic blepharitis
   d. Histopathology — foamy vacuolated cells with
      hyperchromatic nuclei
   e. Treatment — radical excision and radiotherapy
5. Carcinoma of gland of Moll
   a. Very rare
   b. Extramammary Paget's disease
6. Malignant melanoma
   a. Very rare
   b. Arising de novo or as a result of junctional change in a
      naevus

c. Signs
  (i) Itching
  (ii) Bleeding
  (iii) Pigmentary changes
  (iv) Change in size of an existing naevus
d. Types
  (i) Lentigo Maligna — superficial premalignant condition of the elderly
  (ii) Superficial spreading
  (iii) Nodular — occurs only in covered areas, not on face
e. Prognosis — depends on site, depth of invasion (poor if invasion greater than 1.5 mm) and degree of inflammation

Miscellaneous conditions
1. Cyst of Moll
   a. Retention cyst
   b. Clear fluid filled
2. Cyst of Zeis
   a. Retention cyst
   b. White cheesy material

Orbit

ANATOMY

1. Pyramidal, volume approximately 30 ml
2. Constricted anteriorly
3. Maximum diameter 1 cm behind rim (equator of globe in this position)
4. Medial walls parallel
5. Lateral walls perpendicular to each other
6. Medial and lateral walls intersect at 45°
7. Orbital axis 22.5°
8. Anterior opening roughly square
9. Height approximately 34 mm
10. Width approximately 39 mm
11. Depth approximately 40 mm

Walls

1. Roof
   Thin. Made up of frontal bone, lesser wing of sphenoid
   a. Superiorly — frontal sinus, anterior cranial fossa
   b. Anterolaterally — lacrimal gland depression
   c. Anteromedially — trochlear depression (4 mm behind rim). Spina trochlearis in 10% of skulls
   d. Anteriorly — supraorbital notch (1/3 from medial end)
2. Medial
   Very thin (0.2–0.4 mm). Made up of frontal, maxillary, lacrimal, ethmoid and body of sphenoid bones
   a. Medially — nasal sinuses and anterior ethmoidal artery and nerve
   b. Anteriorly — lacrimal fossa (anterior and posterior crests)
   c. Superiorly — frontoethmoid suture (obliterated with age)
   d. Posteriorly — posterior ethmoidal artery and nerve just anterior to optic canal
3. Floor
   Thin (0.5–1.00 mm). Made up of maxillary, zygomatic and palatine bones
   a. Inferiorly — maxillary sinus. Infraorbital foramen 4 mm below rim, 1/3 from medial end

b. Medially — fossa of inferior oblique insertion (inferolateral to nasolacrimal duct)
4. Lateral
   Strongest, no relation to sinuses. Made up of zygomatic bone and greater wing of sphenoid bone
   a. Anterolaterally — temporal fossa
   b. Posterolaterally — middle cranial fossa
   c. Anteriorly — lateral orbital tubercle, 11 mm below fronto-zygomatic suture. Insertion of:
      (i) Lateral palpebral ligament
      (ii) Lateral rectus check ligament
      (iii) Levator aponeurosis
      (iv) Suspensory ligament of globe
   d. Superiorly — frontozygomatic suture (common site for dermoids)
   e. Laterally — zygomatic foramina (zygomatico-facial and zygomatico-temporal nerves)

Contents
1. Globe
2. Orbital fat
3. External ocular muscles
4. Nerves
5. Vessels
6. Lacrimal gland

Superior orbital fissure
1. Approximately 2 cm long
2. Connects orbit with middle cranial fossa
3. Laterally occluded by dura and periorbita

Inferior orbital fissure
1. Approximately 2 cm long
2. Superiorly — greater wing of sphenoid/maxillary bones
3. Inferiorly — palatine/maxillary/zygomatic bones
4. Connects orbit with infratemporal and pterygopalatine fossae
5. Separated from superior orbital fissure by neck of sphenoid
6. Transversed by maxillary nerve
7. Transmits zygomatic nerve, sympathetic fibres and venous anastamosis
8. Largely occluded

Branches of the ophthalmic artery
1. Central retinal artery
2. Posterior ciliary arteries
   a. About 15 short arteries
   b. About 2 long arteries
3. Lacrimal artery

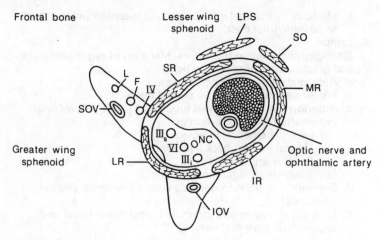

Fig. 1 Superior orbital fissure (schematic diagram)
Key:
Above annulus of Zinn — SOV = superior orbital vein; L = lacrimal nerve; F = frontal nerve; IV = fourth nerve
Through annulus of Zinn — III_s = third nerve (superior division); NC = nasociliary nerve; III_i = third nerve (inferior division); VI = sixth nerve
Below Annulus of Zinn — IOV = Inferior orbital vein
Muscles — LPS = levator palpebrae superioris; SO = superior oblique; SR = superior rectus; MR = medial rectus; IR = inferior rectus; LR = lateral rectus

4. Recurrent branches
5. Muscular branches — anterior ciliary arteries
6. Supraorbital artery
7. Ethmoidal arteries — posterior and anterior
8. Medial palpebral arteries — superior and inferior
9. Terminal branches
   a. Supratrochlear artery
   b. Dorsal nasal arteries

Optic Foramen
1. Transmits optic nerve and ophthalmic artery through sphenoid bone
2. Downward and outward at 36° to the midline
3. Lateral wall 5–7 mm in length
4. Roof 10–12 mm in length
5. Dura adherent to walls
6. Ophthalmic artery inferior then lateral to optic nerve
7. Medially — sphenoid sinus and posterior ethmoid air cells

Periorbita
1. Lines orbit
2. Adherent at sutures and foramina
3. Binds down superior oblique tendon
4. Thickened at orbital rim
5. Divides to enclose lacrimal sac
6. Continuous over superior orbital fissure and inferior orbital fissure

EMBRYOLOGY
1. Ethmoid, sphenoid — from cartilage
2. Frontal, lacrimal — from membrane
3. Maxilla, palatine, zygoma — from first branchial arch

ORBITAL SYMPTOMS
1. Proptosis
2. Diplopia
3. Visual impairment
4. Pain

ORBITAL SIGNS AND EXAMINATION
1. Proptosis
Measure with Hertel exophthalmometer from lateral orbital rim to corneal apex — normal < 20 mm; 2 mm difference between eyes is significant
Types:
    a. Axial — intraconal (dysthyroid commonest)
    b. Nonaxial — extraconal (95% tumours)
Dynamic properties:
    a. Increase with Valsalva manoeuvre
    b. Pulsation
2. Vision
May be impaired due to:
    a. Optic nerve compression due to raised intraorbital pressure (tight septum). Colour vision affected early
    b. Raised intraocular pressure
    c. Exposure keratopathy
    d. Choroidal folds
    e. Pseudohypermetropia
3. Squint
    a. Ocular movements
    b. Forced duction test
4. Palpation
    a. Lumps and local swellings (check lacrimal gland)

     b. Tenderness
     c. Retropulsion
  5. Auscultation
Listen for bruit (e.g. caroticocavernous fistula)
  6. Slit lamp
     a. Tear film
     b. Superior limbic keratoconjunctivitis
     c. Conjunctival vessels — arterialized (dural shunt)
                       — tortuous at muscle insertion
                            (dysthyroid eye disease)
     d. Raised intraocular pressure particularly on upgaze
  7. Ophthalmoscopy
     a. Disc pallor
     b. Disc swelling
     c. Opticociliary shunts
     d. Choroidal folds
  8. General examination

CAUSES OF PSEUDOPROPTOSIS

  1. Ipsilateral
     a. High myopia
     b. Buphthalmos
     c. Orbital asymmetry
     d. Lid retraction
  2. Contralateral
     a. Enophthalmos
     b. Ptosis

CAUSES OF PULSATILE PROPTOSIS

  1. Caroticocavernous fistula
  2. Large frontal mucocele
  3. Meningoencephalocele
  4. Arteriovenous malformation
  5. Neurofibromatosis in children

RADIOGRAPHIC VIEWS OF THE ORBIT

  1. Caldwell view — general view
  2. Waters' view — orbital floor
  3. Rhese view — optic foramen
  4. Lateral view/axial basal view — sinuses

RADIOGRAPHIC FINDINGS IN ORBITAL DISEASE

  1. Orbital enlargement
     a. Tumour
     b. Trauma

2. Bony erosion — benign tumour
3. Bony destruction — malignant tumour (primary or secondary)
4. Hyperostosis
   a. Paget's disease
   b. Meningioma
   c. Osteoblastic secondaries
   d. Fibrous dysplasia
5. Calcification
   a. Phlebolith
   b. Meningioma
   c. Lacrimal gland carcinoma
   d. Retinoblastoma
   e. Foreign body
   f. Calcified parasites
6. Superior orbital fissure enlargement
   a. Carotid aneurysms
   b. Orbital tumours
7. Optic foramen enlargement (asymmetry of > 1 mm)
   a. Optic nerve tumour (e.g. glioma, neurofibroma,
      meningioma)

VENOGRAPHY

1. Not commonly used
2. Performed via frontal or angular vein
3. Outlines superior ophthalmic vein in 3 portions:
   a. Extraconal
   b. Intraconal above optic nerve
   c. Intraconal lateral to optic nerve
4. Apsidal veins connect with inferior ophthalmic vein
5. Inferior ophthalmic vein may not fill
6. Need to compare both sides

ULTRASONOGRAPHY (18 000 Hz)

1. A Scan. — one dimensional; time-amplitude study
2. B Scan. — two dimensional; classical W appearance of scan
3. High reflectivity
   a. Dysthyroid eye disease
   b. Haemangioma
   c. Neurofibroma
   d. Fresh haemorrhage
4. Low reflectivity
   a. Cyst
   b. Mucocoele
   c. Varix
   d. Dermoid
   e. Lymphoma

COMPUTERIZED AXIAL TOMOGRAPHY

1. Plane image parallel to orbitomeatal line
2. Pixel size governs definition
3. Hounsfield scale (−1000 = air, 0 = water, +1000 = dense bone)

CONGENITAL ABNORMALITIES OF THE ORBIT

1. Early suture closure
   a. Oxycephaly — all sutures closed, tower skull; proptosis (50%); visual failure; exotropia
   b. Brachycephaly — coronal suture closure
   c. Crouzon's disease — brachycephaly and maxillary hypoplasia; hypertelorism; shallow orbits; proptosis; exotropia; optic atrophy; irregular dentition; hooked nose
   d. All synostoses — may produce hydrocephalus
2. Primary or secondary under development of the orbit
   a. Mandibulofacial dysostosis — hypoplasia of mandible and zygoma; shallow inferior orbital rim; lower lid abnormalities; antimongoloid slant; prognathism
   b. Hypertelorism — early ossification of sphenoid wings; exotropia
   c. Hydrocephalus — shallow orbits; optic atrophy
   d. Micro/anophthalmos — underdeveloped orbits
   e. Buphthalmos — large orbit

FACIAL FRACTURES AROUND AND INVOLVING THE ORBIT

1. Le Fort I — separation of tooth-bearing part of maxilla from structures above (orbit not involved)
2. Le Fort II — separation of central block of face from skull
3. Le Fort III — separation of face from cranium

BLOW OUT FRACTURES OF THE ORBIT

1. Orbital floor — fracture resulting from blunt trauma
2. Medial wall — seldom in isolation
3. Pure — not involving rim
4. Complicated — involving rim
5. May result in incarceration of orbital contents

ORBITAL FLOOR FRACTURES

1. Clinical features
   a. Suggestive history
   b. Enophthalmos (initially may have proptosis)
   c. Hyper- or hypoaesthesia of infraorbital area
   d. Surgical emphysema

e. Local trauma
f. Limited ocular movements
g. Rise in intraocular pressure on upgaze
h. Nasal bleeding (unilateral)
2. Investigations
   a. Enophthalmos monitoring
   b. Field of binocular single vision, Hess (Lees) screen
   c. Forced duction test
   d. Skull X-ray, Waters' view, Tonogram Findings
      (i) Fluid level in sinuses
      (ii) Hanging drop sign
      (iii) Fracture of orbital rim
   e. CT scan (coronal sections)
3. Management
   a. Conservative — monitor
   b. Surgery — repair at 14 days. Principles:
      (i) Repair defect with bone graft or Teflon plate
      (ii) Squint surgery may be required (inferior rectus recessions + adjustable sutures)
   Indications for surgery include:
      (i) No improvement
      (ii) Enophthalmos > 3 mm
      (iii) Diplopia in primary position
      (iv) Small field of binocular single vision
      (v) Raised intraocular pressure on upgaze

OTHER ORBITAL FRACTURES

1. Orbital roof fractures — associated with sharp objects. Danger of intracranial penetration and retained foreign bodies
2. Trochlear disinsertion
   a. Sharp trauma
   b. Iatrogenic, e.g. whilst approaching ethmoidal artery in treatment of epistaxis

CAUSES OF ORBITAL HAEMORRHAGE

1. Trauma — high risk of visual loss
2. Spontaneous — varices, lymphangioma
3. Iatrogenic — retrobulbar injection

CAROTICOCAVERNOUS FISTULA

1. Causes
   a. Trauma to sclerotic aneurysm (75%)
   b. Spontaneous (25%)
2. Clinical features
   a. Pulsating exophthalmos

    b. Bruit
    c. Diplopia
    d. Pain
    e. Conjunctival chemosis
    f. Increased intraocular pressure
    g. Dilated conjunctival vessels, forehead veins and choroidal vessels (arterialization)
    h. Visual impairment
    i. Optic nerve ischaemia
    j. Intraocular hypoxia (rubeosis)
3. Prognosis — 5% spontaneous cure; 50% vision lost
4. Management
    a. Conservative
    b. Neuroradiological balloon catheter embolization
    c. Internal carotid ligation

ACUTE ORBITAL INFECTIONS

1. Preseptal cellulitis — orbital contents undisturbed
2. Orbital cellulitis
    a. Children usually less than 5 years old
    b. Spread from sinuses
    c. Constitutional features and orbital signs
    d. Usually caused by *Staph. aureus* and Streptococcus
    e. *Haemophilus influenzae* in children less than 3 years of age
3. Orbital abscess
    a. Subperiosteal collections of pus
    b. Complications
       (i) Central retinal artery occlusion
      (ii) Central retinal vein occlusion
      (iii) Optic nerve inflammation
      (iv) Cavernous sinus thrombosis
      (v) Brain abscess

CHRONIC ORBITAL INFECTIONS

1. Causes
    a. Tuberculosis
    b. Syphilis
    c. Fungal (*Aspergillus*)
2. Signs
    a. Irreducible proptosis
    b. Orbital apex syndrome (ptosis; visual loss; internal and external ophthalmoplegia)

ORBITAL INFESTATIONS
1. Cysticercosis (*Taenia solium* larvae)
2. Trichinosis (*Trichinella spiralis*)
3. Hydatid disease (*Echinococcus granulosus*)

DYSTHYROID EYE DISEASE
1. Associations
   a. Hyper/hypothyroidism
   b. Thyroid acropachy, pretibial myxoedema (Graves' disease)
   c. Pernicious anaemia
   d. Myasthenia gravis
   e. Addison's disease
   f. HLA-DR3
2. Aetiological theories
   a. Thyroglobulins and antibodies
   b. Common antigen (orbit and thyroid)
   c. Organ-specific antibodies
   d. Suppressor T cell dysfunction

Ophthalmic features (Werner classification = NO SPECS)
1. *N*o symptoms or signs
2. *O*nly signs, e.g. lid retraction, lid lag, superior limbic keratoconjunctivitis
3. *S*oft tissue swelling, e.g. lid oedema
4. *P*roptosis
   a. Unilateral or bilateral
   b. Acute or chronic
   c. Proportional to septal tightness
5. *E*xtraocular muscle involvement. Most commonly inferior rectus and medial rectus. Infiltrative and restrictive
6. *C*orneal ulceration
7. *S*ight loss
   a. Corneal ulceration
   b. Optic neuropathy
   c. Raised intraocular pressure

Histology
1. External ocular muscles — up to × 8 increased size, infiltration with lymphocytes, necrosis and fibrosis
2. Orbital fat — proliferation and mucopolysaccharide deposits

Investigations
1. Thyroid function — T3, T4, TSH and TRH test (may be hyperthyroid, hypothyroid or normal)

2. Antibodies — including antithyroid microsomal, antithyroid stimulating globulin and other organ specific autoantibodies including those against orbital antigens
3. B scan — enlarged muscles
4. CT scan — enlarged muscles and exclude other orbital pathology
5. Biopsy — rarely used

Management
1. Assess thyroid status. Treatment of thyroid disorder may worsen ocular condition
2. Lubricants
3. Corneal cover
   a. Moist chamber
   b. Tarsorrhaphy (surgically or with botulinum toxin)
4. Guanethidine drops — for lid retraction
5. Intraocular pressure — reduce if raised
6. Steroids
7. Immunosuppressives
8. Radiotherapy (20 Gy)
9. Orbital decompression (3 wall)
10. External ocular muscle surgery and/or injection of botulinum toxin into muscles
11. Lid retractor surgery

PSEUDOTUMOUR

1. Definition. Non-specific, non-neoplastic, polyclonal inflammation affecting any or all soft tissue components
2. Clinical features
   a. Middle-aged females most commonly affected *in adults!*
   b. Types of pseudotumour syndrome
      (i) Bilateral — 30% in children. Associated with polyarteritis nodosa, Wegener's granulomatosis, sarcoidosis and Waldenström's macroglobulinaemia *rare in adults.*
      (ii) Acute myositis
      (iii) Orbital apex syndrome (Tolosa-Hunt syndrome)
      (iv) Orbital and sinus pseudotumour
3. Management
   a. Histological diagnosis to exclude pathology such as lymphoma
   b. Steroids
   c. Radiotherapy

ORBITAL TUMOURS

1. 70% primary
2. 23% direct spread

3. 4% distant spread
4. 3% systemic disease

Vascular tumours of the orbit (commonest primary benign tumours)
1. Capillary haemangioma
   a. Occur in infancy
   b. Anteriorly placed
   c. Dynamic proptosis
   d. With or without strawberry naevus
   e. Initially increase in size, regress by 5 years
   f. Treatment only if amblyopia threatens
2. Cavernous haemangioma
   a. Occur in adults
   b. Slowly progressive, unilateral proptosis
   c. Intraconal with large vascular sinuses within capsule
   d. Surgical treatment
3. Lymphangioma
   a. Rare
   b. May haemorrhage (chocolate cysts)
4. Haemangiopericytoma — very rare

Neural tumours of the orbit
1. Optic nerve glioma
   a. Children, 4–8 years of age. 55% have neurofibromatosis
   b. Optic canal asymmetry in 90%
   c. Fusiform optic nerve enlargement
   d. Benign indolent hamartoma with astrocytic replacement of optic nerve
   e. Management usually conservative
2. Meningioma
   a. Females > males, 40–50 years of age
   b. Primary or from intracranial spread
   c. Early visual loss before onset of proptosis
   d. Slow growing, locally invasive
   e. Fundal signs
      (i) Optic disc swelling
      (ii) Optic disc atrophy
      (iii) Optico-ciliary shunts
   f. Histology — syncytial arrangement of cells with psammoma bodies
   g. Management — conservative or radical excision
3. Neurofibroma
   a. Associated with neurofibromatosis
   b. Proliferation of Schwann cells within nerve sheath
   c. Surgical management

Lymphoproliferative disorders of the orbit
1. Age group — patients usually over 60 years of age
2. Types — range from benign lymphoid hyperplasia (polyclonal) to lymphoma (monoclonal)
   a. Lymphoma — systemic or local disease
   b. Leukaemic deposits ⎫
   c. Plasmacytoma   ⎬ rare
   d. Myeloma   ⎭
3. Management
   a. Biopsy for histological classification
   b. Staging
      (i) General examination
      (ii) Blood count and peripheral blood cell markers
      (iii) Chest X-ray
      (iv) Bone marrow aspiration
      (v) Lymphangiography
      (vi) Whole body CT scan
   c. Radiotherapy (10–30 Gy)
   d. Chemotherapy
4. Prognosis — excellent for local disease

Mesenchymal tumours of the orbit
1. Benign
   a. Fibroma   ⎫
   b. Lipoma   ⎬ all rare, occasional sarcomatous change
   c. Chondroma ⎪
   d. Osteoma   ⎭
2. Malignant
   a. Sarcoma associated with Paget's disease (1%) and orbital radiotherapy for retinoblastoma
   b. Rhabdomyosarcoma
   Clinical features
      (i) Commonest primary malignant tumour in children
      (ii) Average age 7 years
      (iii) Rapid growth of mass in superonasal quadrant
      (iv) Non-axial proptosis
      (v) May have inflammatory appearance
   Pathology
      (i) Embryonal
      (ii) Alveolar
      (iii) Pleomorphic
   Management
      (i) Biopsy to confirm diagnosis
      (ii) Radiotherapy (50 Gy) and chemotherapy
   Prognosis — 90% five-year survival if treated

Lacrimal tumours
1. 50% inflammations and lymphoid proliferations
2. Tumours of epithelial origin   50%
   a. Occur between 20 and 60 years
   b. Non-axial proptosis in 75%
   c. Reduced ocular movements
   d. Astigmatism
   e. Palpable hard nodular mass in 50%
   f. Types
      (i) Pleomorphic adenoma benign mixed cell tumour, 50% of the tumours of epithelial origin
      Features — painless; long history of > one year; local pressure changes on X-ray
      Pathology — must have components of epithelial, myoepithelial and connective tissue; irregular tubular formation; double layer epithelium; myxoid stroma; pseudocapsule
      Management — biopsy contraindicated. Enbloc resection
      Prognosis — good if removed
      (ii) Carcinoma. 50% of the tumours of epithelial origin
      Features — pain; short history of < one year; local bony erosion on X-ray
      Pathology — adenoid cystic; adenocarcinoma; mucoepidermoid
      Management — exclude infection with a two week course of antibiotics. Biopsy if no improvement. Exenteration with removal of bone. Radiotherapy
      Prognosis — poor

Cystic lesions of the orbit
1. Dermoids
   a. Clinical features
      (i) Children
      (ii) Common
      (iii) Painless
      (iv) Slow-growing (increase in size at puberty)
      (v) Upper, outer quadrant commonest
   b. Complications
      (i) Erosion to anterior cranial fossa
      (ii) Ulceration
      (iii) Infection
      (iv) Rupture
      (v) Chronic sinus formation
   c. Management
      (i) Conservative

(ii) Excision — may communicate with an intracranial component. Rupture causes a marked inflammatory reaction. May recur if ruptured. Removal may lead to lacrimal ductule scarring and 'dry eye'
2. Mucocoele of nasal sinuses — may invade orbit

Local spread of adjacent tumours to orbit
1. Nasal sinus carcinomas
   a. Maxillary commonest
   b. Non-axial proptosis
   c. Epiphora
   d. Nose bleeds
   e. Infraorbital anaesthesia
2. Neglected skin tumours
   a. Basal cell carcinoma
   b. Squamous cell carcinoma
3. Extraocular spread
   a. Melanoma
   b. Retinoblastoma
4. Intracranial meningioma
5. Nasopharyngeal carcinoma

Metastatic tumours of the orbit
1. Children
   a. Neuroblastoma 40% develop orbital metastases. Bilateral proptosis and lid ecchymosis
   b. Ewing's sarcoma
   c. Wilms' tumour
   d. Leukaemia
2. Adult
   a. Breast
   b. Lung
   c. Ovary
   d. Kidney

VASCULAR ABNORMALITIES OF THE ORBIT

1. Varix
   a. Commonest vascular abnormality
   b. Non-pulsatile, dynamic proptosis
   c. Phlebolith on X-ray
2. Fistula
   a. High flow (caroticocavernous)
   b. Low flow (dural)
3. Cavernous sinus thrombosis
   a. Cause — results from paranasal sinus inflammation
   b. Features
      (i) Acute onset

(ii) Fever.
(iii) Prostration
(iv) Painful ophthalmoplegia
(v) Conjunctival oedema and congestion
(vi) Proptosis (unilateral becoming bilateral)
(vii) Oedema over mastoid (emissary vein)
(viii) Meningitis and death if untreated
c. Treatment
(i) Systemic antibiotics
(ii) Anticoagulants
(iii) ENT referral

Lacrimal system

LACRIMAL GLANDS

1. Main gland
   Orbital portion makes up 2/3 of gland. Meniscus shaped, situated at superolateral angle of orbit. Fixed to periorbita. 10–12 ductules to upper outer fornix, 1–2 to lower fornix. Palpebral portion lies along ductules, separated from orbital portion by levator palpebrae superioris aponeurosis
2. Accessory glands
   a. Glands of Krause — isolated lobules in upper (40) and lower (6) fornices
   b. Glands of Wolfring — lobules at proximal ends of tarsal plates (3 upper, 1 lower)

Histology
Tubulo-racemose gland, divided into lobules by fibrous septa attached to periorbita. Double layer acini consisting of myoepithelial and cylindrical eosinophilic secretory cells

Blood supply
Lacrimal artery (branch of ophthalmic artery)

Nerve supply to the lacrimal gland
1. Parasympathetic
   Secretomotor. Superior salivatory nucleus via 7th nerve, greater (superficial) petrosal nerve, pterygopalatine ganglion (synapse), zygomatic nerve (5b), and lacrimal nerve (5a)
2. Sympathetic
   Vasomotor. Superior cervical ganglion via deep petrosal nerve, pterygopalatine ganglion (no synapse) and zygomatic nerve (5a)

DRAINAGE SYSTEM

1. Puncta
   Elevated and retroverted. 6 mm from medial canthus. Fibrous ring maintains patency. Increased prominence with age

2. Canaliculi
   2 mm vertical. 8 mm parallel to lid margin. Joins fellow
   forming common canaliculus. Enters lacrimal sac obliquely as
   valve of Rösenmuller. Lined by stratified squamous epithelium
3. Lacrimal sac
   6 × 12 mm. Lying in lacrimal fossa, invested by periorbita.
   Medial canthal ligament anteriorly. Fundus of sac (5 mm) lies
   above and the common canaliculus directly behind the medial
   canthal ligament. Angular vein medially (8 mm from medial
   canthus). Sac slopes laterally and downwards to constriction at
   start of nasolacrimal duct (valve of Krause). Lined by two layers
   of epithelium — columnar and flattened
4. Nasolacrimal duct
   15 mm long. Lying in bony canal formed by maxillary and
   lacrimal bones. Surrounded by rich venous plexus. Passes
   backwards, laterally and downwards, opening under inferior
   concha at physiological valve of Hasner

EMBRYOLOGY

1. Lacrimal gland — ectodermal origin as invagination from
   conjunctiva forming gland. Connective tissue from mesoderm
2. Lacrimal drainage apparatus — formed from buried cord of
   ectodermal cells between frontonasal and maxillary processes,
   later canalizing from above. Canaliculi open at 7th month of
   gestation. Nasolacrimal duct opens soon after birth

TEARS

1. Fornix tears — static pool until full blink provides mixing
2. Marginal tears — brisk flow in meniscus to puncta
3. Precorneal tears — 5–8 μm thick. Stable for 15–40 seconds.
   Ruptures as result of lipid migration to mucous layer,
   particularly in areas of film thinning, resulting in a hydrophobic
   surface. Blink heals rupture

The precorneal tear film

1. Mucin layer (inner layer)
   Glycoprotein layer provided by conjunctival goblet cells
   (holocrine glands), glands of Manz (perilimbal), and crypts of
   Henle (proximal end of tarsal plates). Adsorbed onto microvilli
   of corneal epithelial cells creating a hydrophilic surface
2. Aqueous layer (middle layer)
   Composition varies with age and lacrimal gland disease. 98.2%
   water, 1.8% solids (proteins), pH 7.35. If acid or alkali, produces
   irritation. Glucose concentration low. Hyperosmolarity may
   produce some corneal dehydration. Continuous production
   throughout the day. Basal secretion = 2 μl/min

   a. Causes of reflex aqueous secretion (> 100 μl/min)
      (i) Irritation
      (ii) Yawning, coughing, sneezing
      (iii) Psychic excitation, developing at 4 months of age
      (iv) Photic (bright light)
      (v) Crocodile (aberrant innervation of gland)
   b. Function of aqueous layer
      (i) Oxygenation — provides oxygen to corneal epithelium
      (ii) Protection — dilution. Washing away debris.
           Nonspecific antibacterial agents, e.g. lysozyme and
           lactoferrin. Specific bacterial agents, e.g. secretory IgA,
           IgG
      (iii) Optical — smooth anterior refracting surface
3. Oily layer (outer layer)
   Thin layer of low melting point cholesterol esters and lecithin
   produced by meibomian glands.
   a. Functions of oily layer
      (i) Aids vertical stability of aqueous phase
      (ii) Reduces evaporation
      (iii) Prevents lid margin overflow

Tear drainage
1. Conjunctival sac volume = 35 μl
2. Overflow of margins at 100 μl
3. Between 10 and 50% of tear production evaporates
4. Tear pump
   a. Capillary action into canaliculi
   b. Siphoning action (resulting from the contraction of Horner's
      muscle) drains canaliculi
   c. Pumping action expands sac, sucking tears into sac
   d Sac empties under the effect of gravity

Symptoms of a dry eye
1. Red eye
2. Burning sensation
3. Itching sensation
4. Uncomfortable eye
5. Secondary epiphora in some cases

Ocular examination of a patient with suspected dry eyes
1. Slit Lamp
   a. Meniscus size decreased
   b. Tear film debris
   c. Corneal epithelial filaments
   d. Punctate epithelial erosions, ulcerations
   e. Vital staining with rose bengal 1% (staining of interpalpebral
      devitalized cells and mucus)

2. Schirmer's tests
   a. Type 1 — wetting of Whatman no. 41 filter paper
      (i) reflex: no topical anaesthesia. Normal 10–30 mm
          wetting
      (ii) basic: with anaesthesia
   b. Type 2 — measurement of basal secretion with nasal
      mucosal irritation
3. Lysozyme assay
   Incubation of tears with bacteria (*Micrococcus lysodeikticus*) on
   agar plate for 24 hours. Reduced activity in Sjögren's syndrome
4. Tear osmolarity
   Normal (302 mOsm/l ± 6.3 mOsm/l). Increased in aqueous
   deficiency (343 mOsm/l ± 32.3 mOsm/l)

Causes of aqueous deficiency
1. Congenital absence of gland
2. Riley-Day syndrome (familial dysautonomia)
3. Surgical removal of gland
4. Sensory arc defect (trigeminal nerve defect)
5. Motor arc defect (facial nerve defect, cholinergic blockade)
6. Ductule scarring
7. Ductule destruction, e.g. removal of a lateral dermoid may
   destroy ductules
8. Inflammatory lesions
   a. Primary and secondary Sjögren's syndrome
   b. Mikulicz syndrome

Mucin deficiency

Signs
1. Bitot's spots — interpalpebral conjunctival foamy patches
2. Conjunctival keratinization (xerophthalmia). Lack-lustre cornea
3. Tear break up time — break up of fluorescein-stained tear film
   in less than 10 seconds is abnormal

Causes
1. Vitamin A deficiency
2. Conjunctival cicatrization resulting in goblet cell loss

Causes of an abnormal oily layer
1. Seborrhoeic blepharitis
2. Staphylococcal blepharitis associated with hypersecretion of
   the aqueous component
3. Meibomianitis

Management of dry eyes
1. Artificial tears — cellulose ethers, mucomimetic polymers,
   polyvinyl alcohol

2. Antibiotics
3. Lid hygiene
4. Mucolytic agents, e.g. acetylcysteine
5. Surgery to lid deformities
6. Hydroxypropyl cellulose inserts
7. Punctal occlusion
   a. gelatine rods (temporary)
   b. cautery (permanent)
8. Moist chamber goggles
9. Continuous pumps

WATERING EYES

Causes
1. Hypersecretion
2. Dry eye with hypersecretion
3. Lacrimal pump failure, e.g. 7th nerve palsy
4. Lid — globe incongruity such as ectropion
5. Obstruction of drainage system

Ocular examination
1. Exclude dry eye with reflex hypersecretion
2. Check punctal position and patency
3. Apply lacrimal sac pressure looking for reflux
4. Nasal examination

Tests of the drainage system
1. Fluorescein disappearance test (< 2 minutes)
2. Taste test (saccharin/quinine)
3. Jones' primary test — staining of nasal swab after instillation of fluorescein in fornix
4. Jones' secondary test — if primary test is negative — irrigation of sac with saline. If staining occurs, dye was present in sac. If no staining, lacrimal pump failure is the cause
5. Dacryoscintogram — instillation of ^{99}Tc. Physiological test
6. Dacryocystogram — injection of Lipiodol. Outlines drainage system
7. Probing — elucidates site of block. Therapeutic manoeuvre in distal obstruction of childhood

PUNCTAL OBSTRUCTION

Causes
1. Congenital
2. Senile
3. Cicatrizing disease, e.g. Stevens-Johnson
4. Trauma, e.g. mechanical, chemical or radiation

5. Drug-induced, e.g. practolol, idoxuridine, adrenaline, pilocarpine and Phospholine Iodide
6. Resulting from ectropion
7. Physical, e.g. tumours

Treatment
1. Conservative — astringents, e.g. zinc/adrenaline drops
2. Surgical — lid procedures such as punctal dilation, one snip procedure and ectropion correction

CANALICULAR OBSTRUCTION

Causes
1. Congenital — avoid early surgery
2. Trauma — primary repair with tubing; secondary repair with canaliculodacryocystorhinostomy
3. Infection — Canaliculitis; commonly *Actinomyces israelii* — gram positive anaerobic rod. First treat with antibiotics, then canaliculotomy and debridement
4. Dacryolith — surgery

Surgical treatment
Within 8 mm of punctum — Lester-Jones tubing
More than 8 mm from punctum —
canaliculodacryocystorhinostomy with O'Donoghue tubes
Partial obstruction — insertion of Crawford's tubes or Viers rods

LACRIMAL SAC OBSTRUCTION

Causes
1. Trauma
2. Infection
   a. Acute — painful swelling (dacryocystitis). Treatment with antibiotics and drainage if necessary
   b. Recurrent — dacryocystectomy first; Lester-Jones tubes subsequently
   c. Chronic — results in obstruction and mucocoele formation. Treatment with dacryocystorhinostomy

NASOLACRIMAL DUCT OBSTRUCTION

Causes
1. Congenital — failure of canalization of inferior end of duct, resulting in recurrent conjunctivitis. Treatment with lacrimal sac massage and antibiotics. Probing after 1 year. Rarely dacryocystorhinostomy
2. Trauma — facial fractures
3. Nasal pathology — polyps, antral carcinomas

LACRIMAL GLAND INFLAMMATION

Causes
1. Mumps
2. Glandular fever
3. Suppurative adenitis
4. Extension of conjunctivitis
5. Tuberculosis
6. Sarcoidosis
7. Lymphoma
8. Sjögren's syndrome

LACRIMAL GLAND TUMOURS — see Orbit

LACRIMAL SAC TUMOURS

1. Features
   a. Rare
   b. Painless swelling
   c. Regurgitation of pus and blood via puncta
   d. Outlined with dacryocystogram
2. Histology
   a. Squamous cell carcinoma
   b. Transitional cell papilloma or carcinoma
   c. Adenocarcinoma

Conjunctiva

Conjunctiva

1. Thin membrane lining the conjunctival sac and continuous with the epithelium of the eyelids and cornea
2. Regions
   a. Palpebral
      (i) Marginal — extending from grey line to subtarsal groove
      (ii) Tarsal — adherent to tarsal plates
      (iii) Orbital — folded and loose
   b. Forniceal — reaching behind orbital rim extending behind globe equator
   c. Bulbar — lining sclera, extending to cornea
3. Plica semilunaris — part of medial bulbar conjunctiva; narrow fold producing 2 mm cul de sac
4. Caruncle — at medial canthus; 3 × 5 mm; receiving some insertion of medial rectus

Conjunctival histology

1. Epithelium — stratified non-keratinizing epithelium. Goblet cells are numerous in lower fornix and plica. Melanocytes more numerous at limbus. Regional variations:
   a. Marginal — transitional zone
   b. Tarsal — 2 layers of cells
   c. Bulbar — increasing number of intermediate layers
   d. Limbus — 10–15 layers with basal folding
   e. Plica — 8–10 layers with profuse goblet cells
   f. Caruncle — marginal like epithelium. Fine hairs, lacrimal, sweat and sebaceous glands
2. Substantia propria — deep layers beneath epithelium. Contains blood vessels, nerves, conjunctival glands and immune reactive cells
   a. Adenoidal layer
      (i) Develops by 3 months of age
      (ii) Contains lymphoid follicles
      (iii) Well developed in fornices

b. Fibrous layer — deeper, connecting epithelium to Tenon's capsule

Blood supply of conjunctiva
1. Marginal arcade of eyelid — marginal conjunctiva
2. Peripheral arcade of eyelid — forniceal conjunctiva
3. Posterior conjunctival artery (branch of peripheral arcade) — to within 4 mm of the limbus
4. Anterior conjunctival artery(branch of anterior ciliary artery) — limbus; capillary arcades extend 1 mm into cornea

Nerve supply of conjunctiva
1. Branches of ophthalmic division of 5th nerve
2. Branches of maxillary division of 5th (infero-medial)

Lymphatic drainage of conjunctiva
1. Submandibular nodes
   Drain
   a. medial $\frac{1}{3}$ of upper conjunctiva
   b. medial $\frac{2}{3}$ of lower conjunctiva
2. Preauricular nodes
   Drain
   a. lateral $\frac{2}{3}$ of upper conjunctiva
   b. lateral $\frac{1}{3}$ of lower conjunctiva

Embryology
1. Ectodermal origin
2. Plica semilunaris formed at same time as eyelids
3. Caruncle formed later by separation from lower lid at the time of canalicular formation

FUNCTIONS
1. Tear production
   a. Mucin (goblet cells)
   b. Aqueous (accessory lacrimal glands)
2. Supply oxygen directly to cornea when the eyes are open
3. Defence mechanism
   a. Non-specific
      (i) Mucin clumping
      (ii) Tear production
      (iii) Intact epithelium
      (iv) Rich blood supply
   b. Specific
      (i) Mast cells
      (ii) Leucocytes
      (iii) Mucosal-associated lymphoid tissue
      (iv) Antibodies, e.g. secretory IgA

CONJUNCTIVAL DISORDERS

Symptoms
1. Redness
2. Stickiness
3. Grittiness
4. Photophobia
5. Lacrimation

Signs
1. Discharge
   a. Serous (viral, toxic)
   b. Mucous (vernal)
   c. Mucopurulent
   d. Purulent
   e. Pseudomembranous — strips off leaving intact epithelium (viral, gonococcal)
   f. Membranous — strips off leaving ulcer
2. Conjunctival reaction
   a. Hyperaemia
   b. Oedema
   c. Follicular reaction
   d. Papillary reaction
   e. Haemorrhage
   f. Granulomata
   g. Scarring
3. Associated corneal reaction
4. Lymphadenopathy

Investigations
1. Microscopy (conjunctival scraping)
   a. Gram stain (bacteria and fungi)
   b. Giemsa stain (inflammatory cells, chlamydia and fungi)
   c. Papanicoulou stain (viral inclusions)
   d. Ziehl-Neelsen's stain (tuberculosis)
   e. Fluorescein labelled monoclonal antibody against invading organism, e.g. chlamydia
2. Culture (conjunctival swabs)
   a. Blood agar (fungi and aerobic bacteria)
   b. Thyoglycollate (anaerobes)
   c. Chocolate agar (*Neisseria, Haemophilus*)
   d. Sabouraud's agar (fungi)
   e. Brain heart infusion (fungi)
3. Biopsy (bulbar conjunctiva, not fornix)
   a. Basement membrane disease
   b. Possibly malignant lesions
   c. Sarcoid
4. General examination, e.g. other mucous membranes

Classification of conjunctivitis
1. According to cause
   a. Bacterial
   b. Viral
   c. Fungal
   d. Parasitic
   e. Chemical and radiation
   f. Trauma
   g. Allergic
2. According to exudate
   a. Purulent
   b. Mucopurulent
   c. Membranous
   d. Pseudomembranous
   e. Catarrhal
3. According to onset
   a. Acute
   b. Subacute
   c. Chronic

Bacterial conjunctivitis
1. *Staph. aureus* — purulent
2. *Streptococcus pneumoniae* — purulent and petechial
3. *Strep. pyogenes* — purulent and pseudomembranous
4. *Haemophilus aegyptius* — mucopurulent, epidemic pink-eye
5. Enterobacteriaceae — purulent (Proteus, Klebsiella)
6. Commensals — purulent (*Staph. epidermidis, Neisseria catarrhalis*, Diphtheroids)
7. *N. Gonorrhoeae* — purulent and pseudomembranous
8. *Corynebacterium Diphtheriae* — membranous
9. *Moraxella lacunata* — angular conjunctivitis (Diplobacillus)

Viral conjunctivitis
1. Adenoviral infections
   a. DNA Viruses
   b. 10 of 31 serotypes cause infections
   c. Mild to severe disease
   d. Bilateral follicular conjunctivitis with lymphadenopathy
   e. Pharyngoconjunctival fever (Types 3 & 7). Fever, pharyngitis and keratitis in 30%
   f. Epidemic keratoconjunctivitis (Types 8 & 19). Keratitis in 80%
   g. Keratitis
      (i) Diffuse punctate epithelial
      (ii) Subepithelial
      (iii) Anterior stromal
   h. Investigations
      (i) HeLa cell culture
      (ii) Rising serum antibody titres

    i. Treatment
      (i) Personal hygiene to prevent spread
      (ii) Steroids for severe keratitis
2. Herpes simplex virus and herpes zoster virus
  a. DNA viruses
  b. Follicular conjunctivitis with or without corneal lesions
3. Myxoviruses
  a. RNA viruses
  b. Measles
    (i) Acute catarrhal conjunctivitis
    (ii) Corneal erosions
    (iii) Koplick's spots on caruncle
4. Paramyxoviruses
  a. RNA viruses
  b. Mumps
    (i) Painful dacryoadenitis
    (ii) Follicular conjunctivitis
    (iii) Keratitis
  c. Newcastle disease
    (i) Unilateral conjunctivitis
    (ii) Pneumonitis (spread from fowl)
5. Picornaviruses
  a. RNA viruses
  b. Acute haemorrhagic conjunctivitis
  c. Rapid onset, bilateral
6. Molluscum contagiosum and verruca vulgaris
  a. Chronic follicular conjunctivitis
  b. Associated lid lesions
  c. Superficial keratitis
  d. Pannus

Chlamydial infections

  — Chlamydia trachomatis
  — Intracellular parasites
  — Serovars A, B & C cause trachoma
  — Serovars D–K cause inclusion conjunctivitis
  — Serovars L1, L2, L3 cause lymphogranuloma venereum
1. Adult inclusion conjunctivitis
  a. Features
    (i) Bilateral, acute, mucopurulent
    (ii) Follicular
    (iii) Preauricular lymphadenopathy
    (iv) Chronic course if untreated
    (v) Associated with venereal disease (urethritis, cervicitis)
    (vi) Keratitis mainly in superior cornea
      Types — epithelial
          — subepithelial nummular lesions
          — marginal infiltrates
          — Micropannus

b. Investigations
    (i) Basophilic cytoplasmic inclusion bodies
       (Halberstaedter-Prowazek) on Giemsa staining
    (ii) Monoclonal antibody techniques, e.g. like ELISA
       (enzyme-linked immunosorbant assay) and fluorescein-
       linked antibodies
c. Management
    (i) Systemic and topical tetracycline or sulphonamides for
       a month
    (ii) Investigation of genito-urinary system
2. Neonatal inclusion conjunctivitis *Best with inclusion bodies*
  a. Features
     (i) Incubation 4–5 days
     (ii) Acute
     (iii) Mucopurulent or purulent
     (iv) Papillary, no follicles until 3 months of age
     (v) Superior pannus, conjunctival scarring
     (vi) Systemic infection with — pneumonitis
                           — otitis
                           — rhinitis
                           — gastritis
  b. Investigations
     (i) Ocular ⎫
     (ii) Rectal ⎬ swabs
     (iii) Throat ⎪
     (iv) Ear ⎭
  c. Treatment
     (i) Topical tetracycline
     (ii) Systemic erythromycin (30 mg/kg)
     (iii) Investigation of parents
3. Trachoma — the world's 2nd major blinding condition
                 — 6–9 million people blind (<3/60) from trachoma
                    (1984 WHO estimate)
                 — infection re-infection cycle
                 — secondary infection cycle (*H. aegyptus*)
                 — lack of immunity to infecting agent
                 — predominantly women and children affected
  a. Classification
     (i) MacCallan classification of conjunctival findings:
        Stage 1   — simple conjunctivitis
                        immature follicles
                        incubation = 4 days
        Stage 2a — follicles predominate
        Stage 2b — papillae predominate
        Stage 3   — cicatrizing: trichiasis
                        entropion
                        Arlt's line

Stage 4   — inactive
varying degrees of scarring
ptosis
xerosis

(ii) New proposed WHO grading:
TF — trachomatous inflammation (follicular). > 5
follicles of > 0.5 mm on upper tarsus
TI — trachomatous inflammation (intense).
Inflammatory thickening obscuring > 50% of
large deep tarsal vessels
TS — trachomatous (conjunctival) cicatrization.
Visible white lines, bands or sheets of fibrosis
TT — trachomatous trichiasis.
At least 1 eyelash or evidence of recent removal
CO — corneal opacity.
Obscuring at least part of pupil margin. Causing
vision < 6/18

b. Corneal changes
(i) Epithelial keratitis
(ii) Infiltrates
(iii) Superior superficial pannus
(iv) Herbert's pits (cicatrized limbal follicles)
c. Investigations — basophilic inclusion bodies in conjunctival
scrapings during active disease
d. Management
(i) During active disease. Systemic and topical antibiotics
(ii) Lid surgery for eyelid and eyelash malposition
(iii) Management of dry eyes
(iv) Mass prophylaxis. Hand and face washing. Antibiotics

Ligneous conjunctivitis
1. Features
a. Rare
b. Affects young children
c. Acute onset, chronic course
d. Possibly related to excessive abnormal mucus
2. Pathology
a. Pseudomembrane with development of large amounts of
granulation tissue
b. Late compaction and invasion of tissue
    steroid, mucolytics, cyclosporin gtts.
Granulomatous conjunctivitis
1. Parinaud's oculoglandular syndrome
a. Features
(i) Monocular
(ii) Granulomatous
(iii) Follicles with necrosis and ulceration
(iv) Lymphadenopathy
(v) Fever and malaise

   b. Causes
       (i) Cat scratch fever
       (ii) Oculoglandular tularaemia
       (iii) Spirotrichosis
       (iv) Tuberculosis
       (v) Syphilis
       (vi) Coccidioidomycosis
       (vii) Lymphogranuloma venereum
       (viii) Actinomycosis
       (ix) Infectious mononucleosis
       (x) Rickettsiae
2. Tuberculosis
    Features
       (i) Secondary to extraocular disease
       (ii) Commonly upper tarsal conjunctiva
       (iii) Pedunculated nodules
       (iv) Shallow, indolent, coalescing ulcers
3. Syphilis
    a. Primary — chancre
    b. Secondary — conjunctivitis
    c. Tertiary — gummatous tarsitis
4. Sarcoidosis — conjunctival involvement frequent
    Features
       (i) Nodules (non-caseating granulomas)
       (ii) Fibrosis (dry eye)

Vernal keratoconjunctivitis (VKC)
1. Features
    a. Recurrent, bilateral inflammation
    b. Especially spring and summer
    c. More common in the tropics
    d. More common in children and young adults
    e. Males > females
2. Symptoms
    a. Itching
    b. Lacrimation
    c. Photophobia
    d. Grittiness
    e. Stringy mucous discharge
    f. Ptosis
    g. Itchy skin
3. Signs
    a. Limbal
       (i) Limbal follicles
       (ii) Trantas' dots (eosinophils clumped at apex of follicles)
    b. Palpebral — superior tarsus, cobblestone papillae
    c. Keratitis
       (i) Punctate epithelial keratitis (superior)
       (ii) Epithelial macroerosions

      (iii) Plaque. Non-wetting ulcer, poor healing
      (iv) Subepithelial scarring
      (v) Pseudogerontoxon. ('Cupid's bow' appearance)
4. Pathology
    a. Flat-topped giant papillae (cobblestones)
    b. Hypertrophy of adenoidal layers
    c. Round cell, eosinophil, mast cell infiltrate
    d. Epithelial downgrowth
    e. Goblet cell proliferation
    f. Fibrosis, hyaline degeneration
    g. Alkaline tears and raised tear IgE
    h. Eosinophilia ($\geq$ 2 eosinophils per high power field)
5 Treatment
    a. Topical sodium cromoglycate drops
    b. Lubricants
    c. Mucolytic agents
    d. Topical steroids
    e. Débridement of plaques
    f. Oral antihistamines
    g. Oral aspirin

Atopic conjunctivitis
1. Features
    a. Type 1 hypersensitivity. Commonly to pollens
    b. Acute onset
    c. Lacrimation
    d. Chemosis
    e. Rhinitis
2. Management
    a. Remove allergens
    b. Topical sodium cromoglycate
    c. Topical or systemic antihistamines
    d. Topical steroids
    e. Desensitization

Giant papillary conjunctivitis (GPC)
1. Affects upper tarsal conjunctiva
2. Causes
    a. Contact lens wear (particularly soft lenses)
    b. Ocular prosthesis
    c. Protruding corneal sutures

Primary irritant conjunctivitis *follicular conj.*
1. Chronic follicular conjunctivitis. Causes:
    a. Topical treatments i.e. active ingredients, preservatives
    b. Meibomian secretions
    c. Seborrhoeic blepharitis
    d. Chemical irritation
    e. Actinic keratoconjunctivitis

f – molluscum conj.
g – chlamydia incl. disease.

Phlyctenulosis
1. Features
   a. Type 4 hypersensitivity
   b. Unilateral
   c. Usually affects children
2. Causes
   a. Staphylococci (most common cause now)
   b. Coccidioidomycosis
   c. Candidiasis
   d. Herpetic infection
   e. Lymphogranuloma venereum
   f. Tuberculosis
3. Pathology
   a. Bulbar conjunctival nodules (0.5–3 mm)
   b. At 10 days, infiltration (lymphocytes)
   c. Apical ulceration, resolution by fibrosis
   d. Limbal involvement may produce corneal vascularization
      and blindness
4. Management
   a. Treat primary condition
   b. Topical steroids and antibiotics

Ophthalmia neonatorum
1. Definition: conjunctivitis within first month of life
2. Notifiable disease
3. Types
   a. Chemical, e.g. Silver nitrate. Occurs in first 24 hours after
      drops
   b. Gonococcal
      (i) 2–4 days
      (ii) Purulent, haemorrhagic
      (iii) Corneal ulceration, perforation
      (iv) Management — urgent gram stain looking for gram
           negative intracellular diplococci. Topical and systemic
           penicillin. Parental investigation *or ceftriaxone*
   c. Staphylococcal — 4–5 days
   d. *Haemophilus* — 4–5 days
   e. Herpes simplex
      (i) 5–7 days
      (ii) Type 2 virus
      (iii) Blepharoconjunctivitis
      (iv) Keratitis
   f. Chlamydial — 5–14 days

Chemical injury
1. Acid burn
   a. Limited injury
   b. Proteins denatured

2. Alkali burn
   a. Saponification of lipid
   b. Deep ocular penetration with potentially severe damage and ischaemia
   c. Complications
      (i) Symblepharon
      (ii) Xerosis
      (iii) Corneal ulceration, failure of epithelialization, stromal ulceration, and stromal melt. Late vascularization
      (iv) Uveitis
      (v) Cataract
      (vi) Secondary glaucoma
      (vii) Phthisis
   d. Treatment
      (i) Irrigation
      (ii) Steroids (1st week)
      (iii) Sodium Ascorbate 10% drops
      (iv) Collagenase inhibitors
      (v) Lubricants
      (vi) Symblepharon lysis and prevention, e.g. contact lens
      (vii) Eyelid surgery
      (viii) Keratoplasty later (poor results)

Benign mucous membrane pemphigoid
1. Onset in 6th decade
2. Females more commonly affected
3. Autoimmune disease associated with HLA-B12
4. Features
   a. Skin
      (i) Recurrent vesicobullous lesions in inguinal areas and extremities
      (ii) Scarring lesions over scalp and face
   b. Mucous membranes — nose, pharynx, larynx, oesophagus, anus and vagina scar producing strictures
   c. Ocular
      (i) Bilateral, relentless course
      (ii) Papillary conjunctivitis, pseudo-membranes
      (iii) Subconjunctival fibrosis
      (iv) Aqueous (sicca) and mucus (xerosis) tear deficiency
      (v) Symblepharon. Ankyloblepharon
      (vi) Entropion, trichiasis, lagophthalmos
      (vii) Corneal exposure, opacification, and vascularization
5. Histology
   a. Epithelial thinning
   b. Loss of goblet cells
   c. Keratinization
   d. Subepithelial inflammation and fibrosis

    e. Antibasement membrane antibody on immunofluorescent staining
6. Treatment
    a. Lubricants
    b. Antibiotics
    c. Contact lens
    d. Eyelid surgery
    e. Steroids (topical and systemic)
    f. Immunosuppressants
    g. Keratoprostheses

Steven's-Johnson syndrome
1. Affects young people
2. Causes
    a. Post infections (bacteria, mycoplasma, herpes simplex virus)
    b. Drugs, e.g. Sulphonamides. 25% recurrence on re-exposure
3. Features
    a. Erythema multiforme
       (i) Symmetrical 'target' lesions
       (ii) Extensor surfaces
       (iii) Skin pigmentation
    b. Mucous membranes
       (i) Oesophageal and genito-urinary membrane ulcers and strictures
       (ii) Oral ulceration
    c. Ocular
       (i) Conjunctival ulceration and secondary infection
       (ii) Subepithelial fibrosis and symblepharon
       (iii) Trichiasis, sicca, xerosis
       (iv) Corneal exposure, opacification, pannus
       (v) Visual loss
    d. General
       (i) Arthralgia
       (ii) Fever
       (iii) Sore throat
       (iv) Malaise
4. Histopathology (conjunctiva)
    a. Early
       (i) Epithelial thinning
       (ii) Fibrinous exudate
       (iii) Stromal lymphocytic infiltrate
    b. Late
       (i) Patchy epidermalization (Rete pegs, prickle cells, epithelial thickening, and keratinization)
       (ii) Subepithelial fibrosis
5. Management
    a. Remove causative agents
    b. Steroids

c. Symblepharon lysis, e.g. contact lens
d. Antibiotics
e. Lid and conjunctival surgery
f. Corneal grafts (poor prognosis)

Drugs causing cicatricial conjunctival disease
1. Systemic — practolol (oculomucocutaneous syndrome)
2. Topical
   a. Adrenaline
   b. Pilocarpine
   c. Phospholine iodide
   d. Antivirals, e.g. F_3T

Superior limbic keratoconjunctivitis
1. Affects mainly middle aged women
2. Symptoms greater than signs suggest
3. Associations
   a. Dysthyroid eye disease
   b. Following intraocular surgery
   c. Viral infections
4. Features
   a. Bilateral, chronic
   b. Changes located superiorly on eye
   c. Tarsal papillary hypertrophy
   d. Bulbar conjunctival injection
   e. Limbitis
   f. Filamentary keratitis   DES too hes it.
5. Management
   a. Lubricants
   b. Acetylcysteine drops
   c. Soft contact lens
   d. Check thyroid status

Degenerations
1. Lithiasis — concretions. Resulting from prolonged conjunctivitis
2. Pinguecula
   a. Yellow/white perilimbal plaques
   b. Histology
      (i) Epithelial thinning
      (ii) Elastoid stromal degeneration
3. Pterygium
   a. Wing-shaped fibrovascular overgrowth onto cornea in interpalpebral space
   b. Related to chronic exposure to ultraviolet light and dryness
   c. Histology
      (i) Epithelial thinning
      (ii) Elastoid degeneration

(iii) Fragmentation of Bowman's membrane
(iv) Iron deposition line (Stocker's line)
d. Indications for treatment
  (i) Cosmetic
  (ii) Visual axis threatened
e. Treatments
  (i) Excision
  (ii) Lamellar graft
  (iii) Bare scleral techniques
  (iv) Beta-irradiation
  (v) Thiotepa

'Cystic' conjunctival lesions
1. Simple cysts (serous)
2. Implantation cysts
   a. Surgical
   b. Traumatic
3. Granulomas
   a. Retained foreign body
   b. Suture material
4. Dermoids
   a. Congenitally displaced embryonic epithelium
   b. Occasionally deep connections
   c. May contain hair follicles
   Goldenhar's syndrome
     (i) Bilateral limbal dermoids
     (ii) Preauricular skin tags
     (iii) Aural fistulae, vertebral anomalies
     (iv) Facial and widespread neuromuscular and skeletal anomalies

Conjunctival vascular anomalies
1. Lymphangiectasia — dilated lymph channels
2. Telangectasia
   a. Ataxia-telanigectasia (Louis-Bar syndrome)
   b. Osler-Weber-Rendu syndrome
   c. Sturge-Weber syndrome
   d. Extracranial/intracranial fistula
   e. Irradiation
   f. Mustard gas

Nonpigmented conjunctival lesions
1. Papilloma
   a. Benign, pedunculated
   b. Histology — thickened squamous epithelium
2. Dyskeratosis (leucoplakia)
   a. Epithelial hyperplasia
   b. Keratinization

   c. Elastoid degeneration of stroma with or without
      inflammation
3. Bowen's disease
   a. Intraepithelial carcinoma-in-situ
   b. Commoner at 60 years of age and over
   c. Males > females
   d. Interpalpebral, perilimbal, raised, reddish-grey and
      vascularized lesion
   e. Slow growing and may invade the cornea
   f. Histopathology
      (i) Proliferation of basal cells
      (ii) Loss of cellular polarity
      (iii) Hyperchromatic nuclei
      (iv) Mitotic activity
      (v) Basement membrane intact
   g. Management
      (i) Biopsy
      (ii) Radiotherapy
      (iii) Excision
4. Squamous cell carcinoma
   a. Macroscopically similar to Bowen's disease carcinoma
   b. Stromal invasion occurs
   c. Local and distant spread
   d. Histopathology
      (i) Pleomorphic cells
      (ii) Keratin nest formation
      (iii) Stromal invasion
   e. Management
      (i) Biopsy
      (ii) Radiotherapy
      (iii) Excision
5. Other tumours
   a. Rare
   b. Benign or malignant
   c. Originate from:
      (i) Glandular tissue
      (ii) Connective tissue
      (iii) Vascular tissue
      (iv) Lymphoid tissue
      (v) Peripheral nerves

Pigmented conjunctival lesions
1. Pseudo-pigmented lesions
   a. Blue sclera, e.g. in osteogenesis imperfecta, Ehlers-Danlos
      and Marfan's syndromes
   b. Scleromalacia perforans
   c. Staphylomas

2. Exogenous causes
   a. Argyrosis
   b. Mascara
   c. Adrenochromes
3. Endogenous causes
   a. Addison's disease
   b. Nelson's syndrome
   c. Alkaptonuria
      (i) Autosomal recessive
      (ii) Absence of homogentisic acid oxidase (dark urine reducing Benedict's reagent)
   d. Jaundice
   e. Around perforating arteries
4. Melanin containing lesions (see below)

Melanin containing lesions
1. Epithelial melanosis
   a. Racial (perilimbal)
   b. Primary acquired melanosis (premalignant in Caucasians)
   c. Intraepithelial melanoma
      (i) Superficial spreading — middle or old age; radial growth
      (ii) Lentigo Maligna. (Hutchinson's Freckle) — Elderly; Superficial spread
   d. Secondary
      (i) Exposure
      (ii) Ectropion
      (iii) Trachoma
      (iv) Onchocerciasis
2. Subepithelial melanosis
   a. Congenital
   b. Associated with eyelid pigmentation (Naevus of Ota). These cases may be associated with choroidal melanoma
3. Naevi
   a. Features
      (i) Common
      (ii) Single, sharply demarcated, flat or elevated
      (iii) Usually near limbus
      (iv) Appear in childhood or at puberty
      (v) May increase at puberty or during pregnancy
      (vi) 30% non-pigmented
      (vii) Malignant transition rare
   b. Treatment — excision for cosmesis, irritation or if malignant change suspected
   c. Histology
      (i) Similar features to cutaneous naevi
      (ii) In addition, solid and cystic epithelial inclusions derived from surface epithelium may occur

Cornea and sclera

CORNEA

1. Dimensions
   a. Average diameter 11.5 mm
   b. Thickness 1 mm peripherally, 0.5 mm centrally
   c. Radius of curvature, anterior surface 7.8 mm, posterior surface 6.6 mm
2. Histology
   a. Epithelium — 5–6 cells deep, non-keratinizing, stratified, squamous. Zona occludens and microvilli at surface. Regenerates
   b. Bowman's layer — anterior condensation of substantia propria. Scars with trauma
   c. Substantia propria (stroma) — avascular network of interlacing collagen fibrils, scattered keratocytes, mucopolysaccharide and glycoprotein ground substance, corneal nerves
   d. Descemet's membrane — strong collagenous layer. Resistant to chemicals and infective agents. Readily regenerates
   e. Endothelium — polygonal cell monolayer. Cells cannot regenerate
3. Embryology
   a. Epithelium derived from surface ectoderm
   b. Remainder derived from mesenchyme

Physiology

1. Functions
   a. Light refraction. Cornea 43 D (vs 15 D from lens in situ)
   b. Reduction of oblique and spherical optical aberrations (due to aplanatic surface)
   c. Protection against physical, chemical and infective agents
   d. Transmission of light in 400–700 nm wavelength band
2. Composition
   a. 78% water
   b. 4% mucopolysaccharides
   c. 18% collagen

3. Thickness affected by:
   a. Age
   b. Osmolarity of tears
   c. Intraocular pressure
   d. Integrity of epithelium and endothelium
   e. Drugs
   f. Temperature
   g. Disease
4. Transparency due to:
   a. Relative dehydration
   b. Absence of blood vessels and pigments
   c. Regular arrangement of stromal layers and collagen fibrils
   d. Consistent refractive index of all layers (1.336)
5. Metabolism
   a. Mostly in endothelium, epithelium and stromal keratocytes
   b. Preferably aerobic (can survive 7 hours anaerobically)
   c. Oxygen — mostly derived from tear film, some from limbal capillaries (oxygen gradient from tears to the aqueous)
   d. Glucose — 90% derived from aqueous, 10% from limbal capillaries
6. Permeability
   a. Lipid rich hydrophobic epithelium and endothelium. Good permeability to water and lipids, poor to salts. Hydrophilic stroma
   b. Relative dehydration due to integrity of hydrophobic epithelium and endothelium
   c. Osmotic gradient (aqueous and tears are hypertonic)

SCLERA

1. Tough fibrous envelope composed of collagen and elastin fibres
2. Thickness
   a. 1 mm posteriorly
   b. 0.33 mm beneath recti
   c. 0.66 mm at insertion of recti
3. 12 mm radius of curvature
4. Three ill-defined layers
   a. Episclera
   b. Sclera proper
   c. Lamina fusca
5. Pierced by:
   a. Optic nerve via lamina cribrosa
   b. Vortex veins
   c. Posterior ciliary nerves and vessels
   d. Anterior ciliary arteries
   e. Episcleral veins
6. Embryology — derived from mesencyme

CONGENITAL CORNEAL DISEASE

1. Microcornea
   a. Bilateral
   b. Less than 10 mm diameter
   c. Associated shallow anterior chamber and narrow angle. Angle closure glaucoma
2. Megalocornea
   a. Bilateral diameter more than 13 mm (> 12 mm neonates)
   b. No associated glaucoma
   c. Non-progressive
   d. Posterior subcapsular cataract occurs
3. Sclerocornea
   a. Autosomal recessive or dominant
   b. Non-inflammatory, vascularized, peripheral corneal opacification
   c. Non-progressive
   d. Associations
      (i) Cornea plana
      (ii) Aniridia
      (iii) Mesodermal dysgenesis
      (iv) Microphthalmos
4. Epibulbar dermoids
   Limbal or central

Anterior corneal dystrophies

1. Cogan's
   a. Microcystic, map, dot or fingerprint appearance
   b. Often asymptomatic
   c. Can cause recurrent erosions
   d. Presents in fourth decade
   e. Vision unaffected
   f. Symptomatic treatment
2. Reis-Bückler's
   a. Autosomal dominant
   b. Commonest dystrophy
   c. Typical central honeycomb appearance with progressive scarring of Bowman's membrane
   d. Affects epithelium, Bowman's membrane and anterior stroma
   e. Presents in childhood with recurrent erosions
   f. Vision impaired by teens
   g. Symptomatic treatment, eventually requires graft
3. Meesmann's
   a. Autosomal dominant, onset in infancy
   b. Rare
   c. Clear epithelial microcysts
   d. Vision unaffected

  e. PAS positive material in epithelial cells
  f. Symptomatic treatment

Stromal corneal dystrophies
1. Lattice
   a. Autosomal dominant
   b. Appearance of branching, criss-crossed lines
   c. Initially anterior stroma, later deeper
   d. Presents in childhood or teens. Recurrent erosions
   e. Vision impaired by 30s
   f. Localized deposits of amyloid (stains with PAS and Congo Red, with birefringence)
   g. Eventually requires corneal grafting
   h. May recur in graft 4–5 years after grafting ⟵
2. Macular
   a. Autosomal recessive
   b. Most severe corneal dystrophy
   c. All layers affected (initially superficial)
   d. Greyish macular lesions, initially central
   e. Recurrent erosions in childhood, vision impaired by 30s
   f. Mucopolysaccharide deposition in keratocytes and stroma (stains with colloidal iron and Alcian blue)
   g. Eventually requires corneal grafting
   h. Recurrence can occur in graft ⟵
3. Granular
   a. Autosomal dominant
   b. Relatively mild
   c. Central crumb-like opacities
   d. Initially anterior stroma, later deeper
   e. Present in teens with photophobia or abnormal appearance (recurrent erosions are rare)
   f. Vision often normal or only impaired in 40s
   g. Local deposits of abnormal proteins (stains with Masson's trichrome)
   h. Occasionally needs full thickness graft (recurrence is unusual) ⟵

Endothelial corneal dystrophies
1. Fuch's
   a. Familial tendency (no specific inheritance)
   b. Relatively common
   c. 40–70 year age group; commoner in females
   d. Excrescenses on Descemet's membrane with abnormal endothelial cell morphology
   e. Initially axial and symptomless
   f. Later endothelial decompensation and bullous keratopathy
   g. Treat with hyperosmotic agents, bandage contact lens
   h. Eventually requires full thickness graft

2. Posterior polymorphous
   a. Autosomal dominant
   b. Asymmetrical, vesicle-like lesions in Descemet's membrane, variable morphology
   c. Abnormal collagenous membrane is secreted by the endothelium
   d. Usually symptomless, evident from teens onwards
   e. Occasionally associated with iridoschisis, band keratopathy, glaucoma
   f. No treatment required

Ectatic corneal dystrophies
1. Keratoconus
   a. Unknown aetiology, occasionally familial. Onset in teens
   b. Incidence 1 : 20 000
   c. Thinning and bowing forward of inferior paracentral cornea
   d. Progressive blurring of vision due to irregular astigmatism
   e. Other signs
       (i) Munson's sign
       (ii) Fleischer's ring
       (iii) Vogt's lines
       (iv) Central scarring
       (v) Prominent corneal nerves
       (vi) Oil drop sign
   f. Acute hydrops can occur
   g. Treat initially with hard contact lens, later full thickness graft
   h. Associations
       (i) Atopy
       (ii) Down's syndrome
       (iii) Turner's syndrome
       (iv) Marfan's syndrome
       (v) Ehlers-Danlos syndrome
       (vi) Aniridia
       (vii) Retinitis pigmentosa
       (viii) Ectopia lentis
       (ix) Microcornea
       (x) Non-specific, systemic collagen abnormalities
2. Posterior keratoconus
   a. Rare, non-progressive
   b. Posterior corneal surface has variable sized excavations with no associated scarring
3. Keratoglobus
   a. Rare
   b. Unknown aetiology
   c. Thinning of entire cornea
   d. Irregular astigmatism
   e. Treatment similar to keratoconus

4. Pellucid marginal degeneration
    a. Rare
    b. Peripheral corneal thinning
    c. Irregular astigmatism
    d. Occasional hydrops

CORNEAL DEGENERATIONS

1. Band-shaped keratopathy
    a. Extracellular deposition of calcium and hydroxyapatite in basement membrane, Bowman's layer and superficial stroma
    b. In the interpalpebral zone
    c. Swiss cheese appearance
    d. Associated with chronic uveitis (especially Still's disease and ankylosing spondylitis), hypercalcaemia, phthisis
    e. Treatment
        (i) Bandage contact lens
        (ii) Superficial keratectomy
        (iii) Topical EDTA
        (iv) Lamellar grafting
2. Salzmann's nodular degeneration
    a. Superficial, bluish-white nodules
    b. Hyaline deposits in Bowman's membrane
    c. Vision may be unaffected
    d. Can result from chronic inflammatory conditions such as syphilitic keratitis, phlyctenular keratitis, trachoma, viral keratitis
    e. Associated with aniridia
    f. Eventually may need superficial keratectomy
3. Spheroid degeneration (Labrador keratopathy)
    a. Spherical extracellular deposits of eosinophilic material (degenerative collagen)
    b. In subepithelial cornea (and conjunctiva)
    c. Related to u.v. irradiation
    d. May require graft
4. Lipid keratopathy
    a. Extracellular deposition of lipid
    b. Adjacent to areas of corneal vascularization

CORNEAL INFECTIONS

Bacterial corneal infections
1. Clinical presentations
    a. Keratitis
    b. Keratoconjunctivitis
    c. Hypopyon ulcer

2. Predisposing factors
   a. Adnexal infection
   b. Entropion
   c. Exposure
   d. Dry eyes
   e. Contact lens wear
   f. Other corneal disease, e.g. bullous keratopathy
3. Types
   a. *Staph. aureus/Strep. pneumoniae* produce yellowish, opaque, oval, stromal infection
   b. *Pseudomonas aeruginosa* produces an irregular ulcer, diffuse necrosis, semiopaque surrounding cornea, rapid progression. May perforate
   c. Enterobacteriacae cause shallow ulcer, grey-white suppuration and diffuse stromal opacity
   d. *N. gonorrhoeae, N. meningitidis, C. diphtheriae* are unusual causes. Associated with purulent conjunctivitis. May perforate

Chlamydia trachomatis
1. Adult inclusion conjunctivitis (TRIC)
   a. Serovars D to K
   b. Superficial punctate keratitis in 75%
2. Trachoma
   a. Serovars A, B or C
   b. Superficial keratitis in acute stage
   c. Later superior pannus formation

Adenovirus
1. Common; highly infectious
2. Superficial punctate erosions
3. Subepithelial nummular opacities
4. Follicular conjunctivitis
5. Topical steroids alleviate the keratitis

Other viral causes of follicular conjunctivitis
1. Myxoviruses (measles)
2. Paramyxoviruses (mumps)
3. Molluscum contagiosum
4. Epstein-Barr virus (infectious mononucleosis)

Herpes simplex virus
1. Viral characteristics
   a. DNA virus, usually type I, occasionally type II. Intracellular infection like all viral infections
   b. Diagnosis — EM of affected cells, aspirate from blisters, viral culture, monoclonal antibody staining, serial serum antibody titres

   c. Primary infection — self-limiting periocular vesicles and crusting, follicular and papillary blepharoconjunctivitis

   d. Recurrent infection due to reactivation of dormant virus in trigeminal ganglion or cornea. Causes superficial and stromal keratitis

   e. 5-year recurrence rate — 25% after 1st episode, 50% after subsequent episodes

2. Dendritic ulcer
   a. Epithelial disease *— Active virus*
   b. Early coarse punctate or stellate pattern
   c. Later characteristic branching pattern
   d. Ulcer bed stains with fluorescein, margin with rose bengal
   e. Corneal sensitivity diminished
   f. Anterior stromal infiltrates after a few days
   g. Heals in 1–2 weeks, with scarring

3. Geographic ulcer *— Very active virus —*
   a. Enlarged superficial amoeboid ulcer
   b. Usually in association with topical steroid treatment (without antiviral agents)
   c. All have stromal involvement

4. Trophic keratitis *No virus.*
   a. Metaherpetic disease, not due to active virus
   b. Due to persistent defect in epithelial basement membrane
   c. Similar to recurrent corneal erosions

5. Stromal infiltrative keratitis *← Necrotizing J, K.*
   a. Active viral invasion and stromal destruction
   b. Cheesy, necrotic stromal appearance
   c. Associated anterior uveitis and keratic precipitates
   d. May ulcerate
   e. Thinning and vascularized scarring results

6. Disciform keratitis *No virus usually.*
   a. Type IV hypersensitivity reaction
   b. Typical central epithelial and stromal oedema
   c. Folds in Descemet's membrane
   d. Mild to moderate anterior uveitis, with keratic precipitates
   e. May have surrounding ring of cellular infiltrate and antibody/antigen reaction (Wessely ring)
   f. Reduced corneal sensation
   g. Nebular scarring may result

7. Complications
   a. Uveitis
   b. Glaucoma
   c. Episcleritis
   d. Scleritis
   e. Secondary bacterial infections
   f. Perforation

8. Management
   a. Treat superficial lesions with topical antivirals (acyclovir,

Epithelium !!

trifluorothymidine, idoxuridine, vidarabine) and/or
débridement   —Do not use steroids.
b. Geographic ulcers and disciform keratitis require topical
antivirals usually in combination with topical steroids
c. Trophic keratitis requires lubricant ointments and padding.
May need a bandage contact lens —
d. Topical cycloplegics to relieve ciliary and sphincter spasm
and prevent synechiae

Herpes zoster keratitis
1. Viral characteristics
   a. Varicella zoster (DNA) virus
   b. Previous systemic infection (chickenpox)
   c. Virus lies dormant in sensory nerve root ganglion
   d. Affects older age group and immunosuppressed
   e. Diagnose with EM, viral culture, monoclonal antibody
      staining, serial serum antibody titres
   f. Herpes zoster ophthalmicus accounts for 7% of all shingles
2. General features
   a. Painful, red, vesicular rash, progressing to crusting and
      resolution often with scarring
   b. General malaise, lethargy, depression
   c. Occasional dehydration
   d. Post-herpetic neuralgia
3. Ocular features
   a. Occur in 50%. Ocular involvement more common if
      nasociliary branch of 5a affected
   b. Mucopurulent conjunctivitis
   c. Episcleritis
   d. Scleritis
   e. Keratitis
      (i) Peripheral microdendrites
      (ii) Punctate epithelial erosions
      (iii) Filamentary keratitis
      (iv) Nummular keratitis
      (v) Disciform keratitis
      (vi) Neurotrophic keratitis
      (vii) Mucous plaque keratitis
   f. Uveitis in 50% with segmental iris atrophy
   g. Glaucoma
   h. Ophthalmoplegia
   i. Lid scarring with resultant ptosis, trichiasis, ectropion,
      entropion
   j. May get relapsing keratouveitis
   k. Optic neuritis
4. Neurological features
   a. Cranial nerve palsies

   b. Optic neuritis
   c. Encephalitis
   d. Contralateral hemiplegia (rare)
5. Management
   a. Bedrest, prevention of dehydration, analgesia and general
      supportive measures
   b. Systemic antiviral agents in acute stage (acyclovir),
      especially if patient immunosuppressed
   c. Topical antiviral agents in vesicular stage, e.g. acyclovir
      cream to skin, ointment to eye, idoxuridine paint to skin
   d. Skin emollients in crusting stage and treat any secondary
      infections
   e. Topical steroids if keratitis causes scarring or severe uveitis
      (withdraw slowly as steroid dependency results)
   f. Topical cycloplegics to relieve ciliary and sphincter spasm
      and prevent synechiae

Causes of disciform keratitis
1. Herpes simplex
2. Herpes zoster
3. Trauma
4. Vaccinia
5. Syphilis

Fungal and yeast infections
1. Rare
2. Usually aspergillus, fusarium or candida
3. In immunocompromised hosts; with topical steroids; in trauma
   with organic contamination
4. Suspect in suppurative/necrotic keratitis
5. Identify with Giemsa staining
6. Culture with Sabouraud's agar and brain-heart infusion
   medium
7. Treat fungi with topical 5% natamycin
8. Treat yeasts with topical and oral flucytosine

Protozoan/worm/spirochaete infection
1. Acanthamoeba
   a. Rare, but increasing number of cases in recent years
   b. Predisposing causes:
      (i) Soft contact lenses
      (ii) Swimming in freshwater lakes and 'hot tubs'
   c. Persistent keratitis resistant to treatment with antibiotics and
      steroids. Epithelial breakdown. Ring infiltrate. Hypopyon,
      hyphaema and secondary glaucoma. Severe pain and
      chemosis out of proportion with keratitis
   d. Diagnosis — corneal scraping and histology of recipient
      button. Culture on *Escherichia Coli* or *Aspergillus aerogenes*

non-nutrient agar plates. Staining including Giesma, PAS, calcofluor white and fluorescent antibody
e. Treatment:
   (i) Dibromopropamidine ointment ⟩ _Brolene_
   (ii) Propamidine drops ____
   (iii) Neomycin drops
   (iv) Keratoplasty
   (v) Antibiotics for any secondary infection
   (vi) Steroids ???
   (vii) Treatment of any associated glaucoma
2. Interstitial keratitis
  a. Most common cause is congenital syphilis
  b. Acute stromal keratitis with oedema and vascularization ('salmon patch keratitis')
  c. Accompanying granulomatous uveitis
  d. Resolves to leave a stromal nebula with characteristic 'ghost vessels'
  e. Other causes: tuberculosis, mumps, brucellosis, malaria, onchocerciasis, trypanosomiasis, varicella, herpes simplex

Cogan's syndr → IK, deafness/tinnitus = Rx c̄ steroids to prevent deafness

MECHANICAL TRAUMA

1. Scarring only if Bowman's or deeper layers are involved
2. Recurrent erosions can occur following abrasions
3. Disciform keratitis with blunt trauma

ALKALI INJURIES

1. Alkalis in decreasing order of tissue penetrability and potential damage:
  a. Ammonium hydroxide
  b. Sodium hydroxide
  c. Potassium hydroxide
  d. Calcium hydroxide
  e. Magnesium hydroxide
2. Acute features (up to one week)
  a. Partial or total conjunctival and corneal epithelial loss
  b. Corneal clouding and oedema
  c. Ischaemia from thrombosis of conjunctival, episcleral (and scleral) vessels
  d. If severe, fibrinous uveitis, acute glaucoma or hypotony, thrombosis of iris vessels, cataract
  e. Damage varies with alkali type, pH, quantity, area and duration of exposure
  f. Due to lipid saponification and proteolysis
3. Grading the injury
  a. Grade I — corneal epithelial damage. No ischaemia. Good prognosis (full recovery)

    b. Grade II — cornea hazy but iris details seen. Ischaemia of less than one third at the limbus. Good prognosis (some scarring)

    c. Grade III — total loss of corneal epithelium, stromal haze obscures iris details. Ischaemia one third to one half at the limbus. Guarded prognosis (vision impaired, perforation rare)

    d. Grade IV — cornea opaque obscuring view of iris and pupil. Ischaemia of more than half at the limbus. Poor prognosis (perforation common)

4. Early reparative phase (1–3 weeks)
    a. Regeneration of corneal/conjunctival epithelium (unless grade IV)
    b. Resolution of uveitis (unless grade III or IV)
    c. Corneal neovascularization commences (in grades II, III, IV)
    d. Progressive/recurrent corneal ulceration (grades III, IV)

5. Late reparative phase (after 3 weeks) (Grade II, III, IV injuries only)
    a. Corneal neovascularization and scarring
    b. Corneal ulceration persists or progresses to perforation
    c. Conjunctival and episcleral scarring and keratinization
    d. Symblepharon, entropion, trichiasis
    e. Tear film abnormalities
    f. Neurotrophic keratitis

6. Immediate treatment
    a. Copious irrigation with water, normal saline or buffered solutions
    b. Monitor pH
    c. Removal of solid foreign material and necrotic tissue

7. Further management of grade I/II burns
    a. Topical antibiotics, cycloplegics
    b. 10% ascorbate drops (aid collagen synthesis, scavenger for damaging superoxide radicals)
    c. Daily forniceal rodding (or scleral lenses) to prevent symblepharon
    d. Topical steroids (with caution) for first ten days

8. Further management of grade III/IV burns
    a. As for grade I/II but avoid topical steroids
    b. Topical collagenase inhibitors (cysteine or disodium EDTA)
    c. Early conjunctival and/or corneal grafting

ACID INJURIES

1. Acids in decreasing order of potential ocular damage:
    a. Hydrofluoric acid
       Sulphuric acid
       Sulphurous acid
       Chromic acid

b. Hydrochloric acid
   Nitric acid
c. Acetic acid
2. Acid injuries are similar to alkali injuries but less severe due to self-limiting coagulation of surface epithelium
3. Management is similar to that for alkali injuries

RADIATION INJURIES

1. Thermal burns are similar to acid burns
2. Ultraviolet radiation
   a. Causes a punctate epithelial keratitis
   b. Arises 8–12 hours following exposure ('arc eye' and 'snow blindness')
   c. Resolves completely
3. Ionizing radiation
   a. Initial superficial keratitis
   b. Later stromal disruption due to keratocyte damage
   c. Corneal drying secondary to keratinization of conjunctiva

PERIPHERAL CORNEAL ULCERATION

1. Marginal ulcer *- Staph hypersens. ulcer.*
   a. Initial subepithelial infiltrate with peripheral clear zone
   b. Progresses to small, shallow ulcer
   c. Hypersensitivity reaction to staphylococcal exotoxins
   d. Resolves spontaneously
   e. Topical steroids help
   f. Treat any underlying blepharitis
2. Mooren's ulcer
   a. Rare, unknown aetiology
   b. Chronic peripheral thinning or melt
   c. Painful
   d. Blurring due to irregular astigmatism
   e. Often superior. Can spread circumferentially
   f. May perforate
   g. Frequently unresponsive to treatment
   h. Exclude a predisposing scleritis
3. Terrien's marginal degeneration
   a. Bilateral
   b. Peripheral corneal thinning
   c. Painless
   d. Usually occurs in males over 40
   e. Early yellowish stromal opacities in upper cornea
   f. Slowly progresses to non-staining gutter
   g. Vision may be impaired due to astigmatism
   h. Can perforate
   i. May need tectonic graft

System disorders associated with peripheral corneal ulceration
1. Rheumatoid arthritis (seropositive)
2. Systemic lupus erythematosus
3. Polyarteritis nodosa
4. Scleroderma
5. Wegener's granulomatosis
6. Giant cell arteritis
7. Relapsing polychondritis
8. Acute leukaemia
9. Gold toxicity
10. Bacillary dysentery
11. Syphilis
12. Acne rosacea

CORNEAL DEPOSITS

1. Wilson's disease
   a. Kayser-Fleischer ring (in Descemet's membrane)
   b. 'Sunflower cataract'
2. Mucopolysaccharidoses
   a. Only Hurler's, Scheie's, Morquio's, and Maroteaux-Lamy's
   b. Stromal deposition
3. Verticillata
   a. Vortex pattern of epithelial deposition
   b. In Fabry's disease
   c. In systemic drug therapy
      (i) Chloroquine
      (ii) Amiodarone
      (iii) Chlorpromazine
      (iv) Indomethacin
4. Crystalline deposits in
   a. Cystinosis
   b. Oxalosis
   c. Gout
   d. Gold therapy
   e. Argyrosis
   f. Multiple myeloma
   g. Waldenstrom's macroglobulinaemia
   h. Lymphoma
   i. Schnyder's central crystalline keratopathy
5. Iron deposition
   a. Epithelial
      (i) Keratoconus (Fleischer's ring)
      (ii) Pterygium (Stocker's line)
      (iii) Filtering bleb (Ferry's line)
      (iv) Old age (Hudson-Stahli line)
   b. Stromal
      (i) Siderosis
      (ii) Black ball hyphaema

CORNEAL TOXICITY

1. Preservatives
   a. Whorled pattern of punctate epithelial erosions
   b. Superior pannus and erosions (with thiomersal)
2. Antiviral agents
   a. Inhibit epithelial regeneration
   b. Cause punctate epitheliopathy
   c. Include idoxuridine, acyclovir, vidarabine, trifluorothymidine

ACNE ROSACEA KERATITIS

1. Peripheral vascularization typically in the 4 and 8 o'clock positions
2. Corneal thinning (may perforate)
3. Punctate epithelial erosions in lower two thirds
4. Recurrent epithelial erosions in upper cornea
5. Map/dot subepithelial opacities
6. Ultimate neovascularization and scarring

VERNAL KERATOPATHY

1. Punctate epithelial erosions in upper cornea
2. Vernal ulcer. Painless, circumscribed, oval, located in upper cornea, often with a plaque of exudate and mucus in the base
3. Subepithelial 'ring' scar — due to healed ulcer
4. Pseudogerontotoxon
5. Treat with
   a. Topical steroids
   b. Sodium cromoglycate drops
   c. Acetylcysteine drops
   d. Débridement of ulcer base
   e. Oral antihistamines

EXPOSURE KERATOPATHY

1. Corneal drying
2. Punctate epithelial erosions
3. Can progress to ulceration with infection
4. Causes
   a. Proptosis
   b. 7th nerve palsy
   c. Severe ectropion
   d. Coma
   e. Lid trauma
   f. Ptosis over-correction

NEUROTROPHIC KERATOPATHY

1. Anaesthetic cornea
2. Precise pathological process is unclear
3. Punctate epithelial erosions (especially interpalpebral)
4. Can progress to ulceration
5. Causes
   a. Herpes zoster ophthalmicus
   b. Herpes simplex
   c. Trigeminal nerve damage
   d. Diabetes mellitus
   e. Leprosy
   f. Familial dysautonomia
   g. Anhidrotic ectodermal dysplasia
   h. Congenital insensitivity to pain

KERATOMALACIA

1. Corneal melt with xerosis
2. Occurs with vitamin A deficiency
3. Conjunctival keratinization and drying
4. Increased incidence of infection
5. Ulceration and perforation
6. Other causes
   a. Scleroderma
   b. Wegener's granulomatosis
   c. Cytomegalovirus
   d. Rheumatoid arthritis

EPISCLERITIS

1. Features
   a. Inflammation of episclera and overlying conjunctiva
   b. Nodular or diffuse
   c. Benign and self-limiting
   d. More common in young adults. Males = Females
   e. Mild ache, tenderness, burning
   f. Occasionally associated with systemic disease, e.g. Herpes zoster ophthalmicus, rheumatoid arthritis and gout
2. Treatment
   a. Topical steroids and/or oxyphenbutazone
   b. Systemic non-steroidal anti-inflammatory agents

SCLERITIS   _No topical sterods! → perf._

1. Less common but more serious than episcleritis
2. Often very painful
3. Especially affects older women

Anterior scleritis
1. Diffuse non-necrotizing
   a. Segmented or widespread inflammation of anterior sclera
   b. Oedema with distortion of deep vascular plexus
   c. Treat with oral indomethacin/oxyphenbutazone
2. Nodular non-necrotizing
   a. Focal scleral inflammation and oedema
   b. Nodule is immobile
   c. Treat with oral indomethacin/oxyphenbutazone
3. Necrotizing, without inflammation
   a. Scleromalacia perforans
   b. Occurs in sero-positive rheumatoid arthritis
   c. Painless scleral thinning with marked ischaemia
   d. Seldom perforate
   e. Treatment is difficult
4. Necrotizing, with inflammation
   a. Progressive, red and painful
   b. Vascular sludging and occlusion
   c. Focal or diffuse
   d. Associated anterior uveitis
   e. Scleral thinning
   f. 25% 5-year mortality from associated disease
   g. Severe complications, e.g. sclerosing keratitis, peripheral corneal melts, cataract, glaucoma
   h. Treat with high dose systemic steroids, sometimes in combination with immunosuppressive drugs, e.g. azathioprine, cyclophosphamide
   i. Subconjunctival steroids contraindicated

Posterior scleritis
1. Features
   a. Thickened and inflamed posterior sclera
   b. Anterior segment may be unaffected
   c. Easily missed
   d. May have ocular pain or may be painless
   e. Exudative retinal detachment
   f. Thickened posterior sclera (diffuse or focal)
   g. Choroidal folds
   h. Posterior vitritis, disc and macular oedema
   i. Uveal effusion syndrome
   j. Proptosis
   k. Ocular myositis with opthalmoplegia
   l. Usually no associated systemic disorder
2. Investigations — CT scan or ultrasound B-scan may help diagnosis because of thickened sclera
3. Treatment — high dose systemic steroids or immunosuppressive drugs

Systemic diseases associated with scleritis
1. Herpes zoster ophthalmicus*
2. Rheumatoid arthritis*
3. Systemic lupus erythematosus
4. Polyarteritis nodosa
5. Wegener's granulomatosis
6. Dermatomyositis
7. Sarcoid
8. Behçet's syndrome
9. Ankylosing spondylitis
10. Crohn's disease
11. Ulcerative colitis
12. Gout

Uveitis and endophthalmitis

UVEITIS

Nomenclature
Uveitis — inflammation of the uveal tract
Anterior uveitis — mainly iris (iritis) and ciliary body (cyclitis)
  inflammation, e.g. in ankylosing spondylitis
Posterior uveitis — mainly choroidal inflammation (choroiditis), e.g.
  in toxoplasmosis
Panuveitis — inflammation of all parts of the uveal tract, e.g.
  sympathetic ophthalmia

Symptoms
1. Photophobia
2. Pain (deep ocular pain) worsened by accommodation
3. Reflex lacrimation
4. Reduced visual acuity
5. 'Floaters'

Anterior segment signs
1. Ciliary injection (circumcorneal blush from branches of anterior
   ciliary arteries and ciliary efferent veins from ciliary venous
   plexus)
2. Conjunctival and episcleral injection (severe anterior uveitis)
3. Small pupils (iris sphincter spasm)
4. Flare in anterior chamber (turbid aqueous humour)
5. Inflammatory cells in anterior chamber
6. Inflammatory cell on endothelium ('keratic precipitates' which
   are described as 'mutton-fat' if large with waxy or fatty
   appearance)
7. Iris nodules
   a. Koeppe (pupil margin)
   b. Busacca (anterior iris)
8. Hypopyon
9. Dilated iris vessels, occasionally new vessels (rubeosis)
10. Synechiae
   a. Posterior (iris adhesions to lens) → seclusio pupillae

(complete adhesion) may lead to obstruction of aqueous flow through pupil, resulting in 'iris bombé' and angle closure glaucoma
  b. Anterior (iris adhesions to drainage angle and cornea)
11. Iris atrophy
12. Band keratopathy $\Big\}$ longstanding uveitis
13. Cataract

Posterior segment signs
 1. Vitreous cells
 2. Vitreous membranes and opacities
 3. Inflammatory exudates ('snowballs')
 4. Vasculitis — opacification around vessels
   a. Sheathing (whole vessel)
   b. Cuffing (segment of vessel)
 5. Exudates
   a. Cottonwool spot (ischaemia)
   b. 'Candlewax drippings' (greasy appearance)
 6. Retinitis — dull, greyish appearance to retina
 7. Pigmentary changes — hypo- and hyperpigmentation due to inflammation in retinal pigment epithelium
 8. Choroiditis
   a. Focal $\Big\}$ Difficult to distinguish from retinitis without
   b. Multifocal fluorescein angiography
   c. Diffuse
 9. Choroidal detachment
10. Neovascularization (if ischaemia prominent)
11. Macular oedema
12. Optic disc swelling and atrophy

Classification
 1. Idiopathic (largest group)   ⌐RF⊖
 2. Associated with systemic disease (particularly seronegative arthritides)
   a. Ankylosing spondylitis B27
   b. Reiter's syndrome B27
   c. Psoriatic arthritis B27
   d. Inflammatory bowel disease
   e. Juvenile chronic arthritis ⌐ ANA⊕
   f. Sarcoid
   g. Behçet's syndrome B5
 3. Infectious causes
   a. Bacterial
     (i) Tuberculosis
     (ii) Syphilis
     (iii) Gonorrhoea
     (iv) Leprosy

  b. Viral
   (i) Herpes simplex
   (ii) Herpes zoster
   (iii) Cytomegalovirus
   (iv) Measles
  c. Fungal
   (i) Candidiasis
   (ii) Coccidioidomycosis
   (iii) Presumed ocular histoplasmosis syndrome
  d. Infestations
   (i) Toxoplasmosis
   (ii) Toxocara → pan uveitis – panophthalmitis.
   (iii) Onchocerciasis
4. Specific uveitis entities
  a. Fuch's heterochromic cyclitis
  b. Vogt-Koyanagi-Harada syndrome
  c. Sympathetic ophthalmia
  d. Bird shot retinochoroidopathy HLA-A29.
  e. Acute multifocal placoid pigment epitheliopathy
  f. Serpiginous choroidopathy
  g. Bilateral acute retinal necrosis
5. Lens induced
  a. Phacoanaphylactic uveitis
  b. Phacotoxic uveitis
6. Masquerade syndromes
  a. Reticulum cell sarcoma –60–70y/o, tap, LP, rad brain yellow choroid spots
  b. Melanoma
  c. Retinoblastoma

General signs and symptoms
1. Joint problems
  a. Ankylosing spondylitis
  b. Still's disease
  c. Reiter's syndrome
  d. Inflammatory bowel disease
  e. Behçet's syndrome
  f. Whipple's disease
  g. Sarcoid
  h. Leprosy
  i. Metastatic gonococcal disease
2. Diarrhoea
  a. Inflammatory bowel disease
  b. Whipple's disease
3. 'Flu-like' illness
  a. Toxoplasmosis
  b. Leptospirosis
  c. Histoplasmosis

4. Jaundice
   a. Leptospirosis
   b. Inflammatory bowel disease
5. Liver enlargement
   a. Toxocariasis
   b. Cytomegalovirus
   c. Toxoplasmosis
6. Central nervous system involvement
   a. TB meningitis
   b. Vogt-Koyanagi-Harada syndrome
   c. Congenital toxoplasmosis
   d. Congenital cytomegalovirus
   e. Behçet's disease
   f. Reticulum cell sarcoma
7. Skin rash
   a. Secondary syphilis
   b. Sarcoid
   c. Behçet's disease
   d. Psoriasis
   e. Reiter's syndrome
   f. Vogt-Koyanagi-Harada syndrome
   g. Histoplasmosis
8. Erythema nodosum
   a. Sarcoid
   b. Tuberculosis
   c. Inflammatory bowel disease
   d. Histoplasmosis
9. Chest symptoms
   a. Tuberculosis
   b. Sarcoid
10. Urinary disorders
    a. Reiter's syndrome
    b. Metastatic gonococcal disease
    c. Behçet's syndrome
11. Mouth ulcers
    a. Behçet's syndrome
    b. Reiter's syndrome
    c. Herpes simplex
    d. Inflammatory bowel disease

Grading of uveitis

Conditions resembling anterior uveitis
1. Microhyphaema
2. Pigment in the anterior chamber (often after mydriasis)
3. Malignant lymphomas, leukaemia or reticulum cell sarcoma
4. Retinoblastoma
5. Pseudoexfoliation of the lens capsule

Table 1. Cells (Slit lamp beam width 1 mm, length 3 mm; cells counted within this field)

Grade	Cells per field
0	0
+	1–10
++	11–20
+++	21–50
++++	> 50

Table 2. Flare (To grade flare, same setting on slit lamp as for counting cells)

Grading of flare	Description
0	Complete absence
+	Faint = barely detectable
++	Moderate = iris and lens details clear
+++	Marked = iris and lens details hazy
++++	Intense = fibrinous, aqueous

Table 3. Vitritis

Grade	Description
0	Clear vitreous
+	Diffuse scattered opacities, fundal view unimpaired
++	Moderate scattered opacities, fundal detail somewhat obscured
+++	Many opacities, marked blurring of fundal details
++++	Dense opacities, no fundus views

SYSTEMIC DISORDERS ASSOCIATED WITH UVEITIS

Ankylosing spondylitis
Affects young men. 90% HLA-B27 positive
1. General features
   a. Arthritis — sacro-iliac joints and peripheral joints
   b. Heart — aortic incompetence
   c. Colitis (10%)
   d. Lungs — apical fibrosis and restricted chest expansion
2. Ocular features
   a. Acute anterior uveitis. Recurrent attacks in 40%
   b. Episcleritis
   c. Scleritis

Reiter's syndrome
Triad of conjunctivitis, urethritis and arthritis 70% patients HLA-B27
positive. Males >> Females
1. General features
   a. Urethritis (nonspecific)
   b. May follow dysentery
   c. Arthritis — knees, sacro-iliac joints
   d. Plantar fasciitis and Achilles tendinitis
   e. Keratoderma blenorrhagia on feet and hands
   f. Circinate balanitis
   g. Painless mouth ulcers
2. Ocular features
   a. Mucopurulent conjunctivitis
   b. Keratitis with anterior stromal infiltrates
   c. Acute anterior uveitis (30%)

Psoriatic arthritis
Increased incidence in patients with HLA-B17 and HLA-B27
1. General features
   a. Arthritis usually affecting hands, feet and sacro-iliac joints.
      Occurs in 5% of patients with psoriasis
   b. Psoriatic skin and nail changes ~ p13
2. Ocular features
   a. Conjunctivitis
   b. Acute anterior uveitis
   c. Dry eyes

Inflammatory bowel disease
1. General features
   a. Arthritis
   b. Erythema nodosum
   c. Hepatitis
   d. Sclerosing cholangitis
   e. Pyoderma gangraenosum
2. Ocular features
   a. Conjunctivitis
   b. Keratoconjunctivitis sicca
   c. Keratoconjunctivitis
   d. Episcleritis and scleritis
   e. Anterior uveitis
   f. Retinal oedema
   g. Orbital cellulitis
   h. Optic neuritis

Juvenile chronic arthritis   Rx- topical steroids
Seronegative arthritis in patients < 16 years of age
1. General features
   a. Arthritis — pauciarticular if less than 5 joints affected

b. Fever
c. Lymphadenopathy
d. Maculopapular rash
e. Hepatosplenomegaly
f. Myocarditis

} 30% of children with JCA
present with these systemic
features

2. Ocular features _ White eye !!!
  a. Chronic anterior uveitis (usually bilateral). Risk features:
     (i) Pauciarticular arthritis
     (ii) Female with anti-nuclear antibodies
  b. Secondary glaucoma (20%)
  c. Cataract (40%)
  d. Secondary band keratopathy (40%)

Causes of anterior uveitis in childhood
1. Juvenile chronic arthritis
2. Juvenile ankylosing
   spondylitis

} these account for the majority
of cases

3. Psoriatic arthritis
4. Reiter's syndrome
5. Behçet's syndrome
6. Vogt-Koyanagi-Harada syndrome
7. Sarcoidosis
8. Idiopathic iridocyclitis
9. Heterochromic cyclitis
10. Pars planitis

Sarcoid
A multisystem granulomatous disease of unknown aetiology.
Usually affects young adults. Females > Males
1. Presentations
  a. Lofgren's syndrome
     (i) Acute onset
     (ii) Hilar lymphadenopathy
     (iii) Erythema nodosum
     (iv) Anterior uveitis
     (v) Arthralgia
  b. Mikulicz's syndrome
     (i) Lacrimal and parotid gland swelling
     (ii) Sicca syndrome
     (iii) Causes — sarcoidosis
                   — tuberculosis
                   — lymphoma
                   — leukaemia
  c. Heerfordt's syndrome
     (i) Parotid gland enlargement
     (ii) Fever
     (iii) Anterior uveitis
     (iv) Facial nerve palsy

2. General features
   a. Lungs
      (i) Hilar lymphadenopathy
      (ii) Diffuse fibrosis
   b. Skin
      (i) Lupus pernio
      (ii) Erythema nodosum
   c. Bones and joints
      (i) Arthralgia
      (ii) Cystic bony lesions in phalanges
   d. Visceral organs — hepatosplenomegaly
   e. Nervous system — peripheral neuropathy and cranial nerve lesions
   f. Endocrine — diabetes insipidus, hypercalcaemia
3. Ocular features
   a. Eyelids may be involved by purple sarcoid indurating rash (lupus pernio)
   b. Band keratopathy
   c. Lacrimal gland infiltration with enlargement
   d. Conjunctival follicles
   e. Episcleritis and scleritis with nodules
   f. Anterior uveitis
      (i) Acute — particularly in Lofgren's syndrome
      (ii) Chronic — classically of granulomatous type with mutton fat keratic precipitates
   g. Secondary cataracts and glaucoma
   h. Choroiditis with yellow or white nodules
   i. Retinal periphlebitis with candlewax retinal exudates
   j. Retinal neovascularization
   k. Pars planitis
   l. Choroidal granulomas
   m. Optic nerve granuloma

Behçet's disease
Triad of oral ulceration, genital ulceration and inflammatory eye lesions. Males > Females. Commoner in Japan and the Mediterranean. Increased prevalence of HLA-B5
1. General features
   a. Oral ulceration
   b. Genital ulceration
   c. Skin lesions including erythema nodosum
   d. Arthritis
   e. Thrombophlebitis
   f. Large vessel occlusion
   g. Gastrointestinal — pain, diarrhoea, constipation and ulceration
   h. Meningoencephalitis

2. Ocular features
   a. Anterior uveitis (sometimes with hypopyon)
   b. Conjunctivitis
   c. Keratitis
   d. Episcleritis
   e. Retinal vasculitis with retinal infarction
   f. Vasodilatation causing retinal oedema and macular oedema
   g. Retinal exudates in the outer retinal layers

INFECTIONS

Tuberculosis
Disease caused by infection with *Mycobacterium tuberculosis*
Ocular features
   a. Lupus vulgaris on the eyelids
   b. Ectropion from scarring around sinuses associated with
      discharging orbital lesions
   c. Conjunctiva
      (i) Phlyctenular conjunctivitis
      (ii) Primary conjunctival tuberculosis
   d. Keratitis
   e. Scleritis
   f. Lacrimal gland involvement
   g. Orbital periostitis
   h. Granulomatous panuveitis (ciliary body and iris nodules)
   i. 2° glaucoma and cataract
   j. Choroidoretinal plaque or nodule (tuberculoma)
   k. Non-rhegmatogenous retinal detachment
   l. Cranial nerve palsies (basal meningitis)

Acquired syphilis
Disease caused by infection with *Treponema pallidum*
1. Stages
   a. Primary — characterized by ulcerating primary lesion
      (chancre)
   b. Secondary
      (i) Maculopapular rash
      (ii) Lymphadenopathy
      (iii) Fever
      (iv) Malaise
      (v) Condylomata lata
      (vi) Hepatitis
      (vii) Periostitis
   c. Tertiary — local tissue destruction by chronic inflammation
      in any part of the body (gummata)
      (i) CNS — meningoencephalitis

          — general paralysis of the insane
          — tabes dorsalis
   (ii) CVS — aortic aneurysm
          — aortic incompetence
2. Ocular features
  a. Hyperaemic changes in superficial vascular loops of the iris (transient roseolae)
  b. Iris papules and gummata (yellow-red nodules)
  c. Panuveitis resistant to treatment
  d. Choroidoretinitis (localized or diffuse). May mimic retinitis pigmentosa
  e. Optic neuritis or optic atrophy
  f. Argyll Robertson pupils

Congenital syphilis
1. General features
  a. Death in utero or perinatally
  b. Inflammation of internal organs
  c. Dental abnormalities (Hutchinson's teeth)
  d. Facial deformities including 'saddle' nose
2. Ocular features
  a. Interstitial keratitis (keratouveitis) between 5 and 25 years of age. New vessels meet in centre of cornea ('salmon patch'). Vessels then atrophy ('ghost' vessels)
  b. Anterior uveitis in association with keratitis
  c. Dislocated lens
  d. Argyll Robertson pupils
  e. Optic atrophy
  f. Choroidoretinitis
    (i) Diffuse ('salt-and-pepper' fundus)
    (ii) Focal

Leprosy
Chronic granulomatous infection caused by *Mycobacterium leprae*. A spectrum of disease depending on cellular immunity to infecting organism, from tuberculous leprosy (high immunity) to lepromatous leprosy (low immunity)
Ocular features
  a. Lids — lagophthalmos, madarosis, blepharochalasis, nodules, trichiasis, entropion and ectropion and reduced blinking
  b. Lacrimal — acute and chronic dacryocystitis
  c. Cornea — anaesthesia, exposure keratopathy, band keratopathy, corneal leproma, interstitial keratitis, thickened corneal nerves and superficial stromal keratitis
  d. Sclera — episcleritis, scleritis, staphyloma and nodules

  e. Iris — miosis, acute and chronic iritis leading to synechiae, seclusio pupillae, cataract, glaucoma, iris atrophy, iris pearls and leproma
  f. Ciliary body — hypotonia, phthisis and loss of accommodation
  g. Fundus — peripheral choroidal lesions, retinal vasculitis

Cytomegalovirus disease (in immunosuppressed host)
  Ocular features
  a. Anterior uveitis
  b. Retinal oedema and necrosis
  c. Multiple haemorrhages
  d. Microaneurysms
  e. Vascular sheathing
  f. Vitreous opacification and retinal detachment
  g. Optic nerve head mass and optic atrophy
  h. Widespread retinitis and haemorrhages ('Tomato sauce and salad dressing' fundus)

Measles (rubeola)
  Myxovirus
  Ocular features
  a. Keratoconjunctivitis. Blinding disease in malnourished patients with vitamin A deficiency
  b. Retinal oedema
  c. Vascular attenuation
  d. Macular star

Subacute sclerosing panencephalitis (follows measles)
  1. General features
    a. Personality or behavioural changes
    b. Dementia
    c. Seizures
    d. Myoclonus
  2. Ocular features (50%)
    a. Macular or paramacular choroidoretinitis
    b. Pigmentary changes with bone corpuscle configuration
    c. Papilloedema
    d. Optic atrophy
    e. Nystagmus
    f. Cortical blindness

Candidiasis
  1. Occurs in compromised host
    a. Immunosuppressants, steroids
    b. Drug addicts using intravenous injections
    c. Long-term indwelling catheters

2. Ocular features
   a. Anterior uveitis
   b. Retinal haemorrhage and perivascular sheathing
   c. Choroidoretinitis starts with white fluffy lesions ('Puff-balls'). These lesions may be joined by opaque vitreous strands giving rise to the 'string-of-pearls' sign. Proceeds to:
   d. Vitreous abscess formation

Presumed ocular histoplasmosis syndrome (POHS)
Infection caused by fungus *Histoplasma capsulatum*. Endemic in certain river valleys between 45° north and 45° south. Seen in patients with no clinical or serological evidence of histoplasma infection, hence 'presumed' label. Higher prevalence of HLA-B7
Ocular features
   a. Multifocal atrophic choroidal lesions
   b. Peripapillary atrophy
   c. Disciform maculopathy
   d. Streaks of chorioretinal atrophy in the peripheral fundus

Congenital toxoplasmosis
Caused by infection of fetus with obligate intracellular protozoan *Toxoplasma gondii*
1. General features
   a. Stillborn child
   b. CNS damage
      (i) Mentally retarded
      (ii) Convulsions
      (iii) Hydrocephalus
      (iv) Intracranial calcification
2. Ocular features
   a. Anterior uveitis — may be granulomatous
   b. Vitritis
   c. Focal retinitis
   d. Juxtapapillary choroiditis
   e. Optic neuritis
   f. Choroidoretinal scars

Toxocariasis
Caused by infection with *Toxocara canis* and *catis*. Acquired by ingestion of ova.
1. General features
   a. Visceral larva migrans
      (i) Disseminated larvae
      (ii) Fever
      (iii) Lymphadenopathy
      (iv) Hepatomegaly
      (v) Pneumonitis
      (vi) Eosinophilia

b. Subclinical (most of the cases with ocular involvement have subclinical disease)
2. Ocular features
    a. Peripheral retinal granuloma
    b. Localized posterior pole granuloma
    c. Chronic destructive endophthalmitis

Onchocerciasis
Due to infection with filarial nematode *Onchocerca volvulus*. An estimated 40 million people affected (2 million blind). Transmitted by black fly of genus *Simulium* which breeds in fast flowing rivers
1. General features
    Skin — nodules, lichenification and depigmentation. Large folds of skin ('hanging groins'). Erysipelas type or papular rash.
2. Ocular features
    a. Lids — skin nodules and depigmentation
    b. Cornea — sclerosing keratitis. Microfilariae may occasionally be seen in the anterior chamber if patient has been in the dark
    c. Sclera — scleritis
    d. Iris — chronic iridocyclitis
    e. Cataract and glaucoma
    f. Fundus — choroidoretinitis. Optic atrophy (main cause of blindness)

SPECIFIC UVEITIS ENTITIES

Pars planitis
Usually affects young adults. Both eyes involved in 80%. Females > Males
1. Symptoms
    a. Floaters
    b. Impaired vision
2. Signs
    a. Light flare with a few keratitic precipitates
    b. Anterior vitritis
    c. White exudates near the ora serrata (snowballs). Exudates may coalesce to form a snowbank
    d. Mild periphlebitis
3. Complications
    a. Retrolenticular cyclitic membrane
    b. Vitreous haemorrhage
    c. Tractional retinal detachment
    d. Macular oedema
4. Differential diagnosis
    a. Sarcoidosis
    b. Toxoplasmosis
    c. Peripheral toxocara

d. Syphilis
e. Multiple sclerosis

Fuchs' heterochromic cyclitis
Affects one eye of young adults, but bilateralism in up to 80% with long-term follow up
1. Symptoms
   Usually blurred vision from cataract or vitreous opacity
2. Signs
   a. Small keratic precipitates spread diffusely all over the endothelium
   b. Only a few cells and faint flare in the anterior chamber
   c. No posterior synechiae
   d. Heterochromia
   e. Abnormal blood vessels in the anterior chamber angle which may bleed on gonioscopy and during cataract surgery
   f. Secondary open angle glaucoma
   g. Posterior subcapsular cataract
3. Other causes of heterochromia
   a. Idiopathic
   b. Inherited
   c. Trauma
   d. Inflammation
   e. Retained metallic intraocular foreign body
   f. Congenital Horner's syndrome
   g. Melanoma
   h. Waardenburg's syndrome (heterochromia iridis, telecanthus, white forelock and congenital deafness)
   i. Parry-Romberg syndrome (heterochromia iridis, Horner's syndrome, oculomotor palsies, nystagmus and facial hemiatrophy)
   j. Glaucomatocyclitic crisis

Vogt-Koyanagi-Harada syndrome
Occurs between the ages of 30 and 50 years. Much more common in Japanese patients
1. Cutaneous features
   a. Alopecia
   b. Vitiligo
   c. Whitening of eyelashes (poliosis)
2. CNS features
   a. Meningeal irritation with headache and neck stiffness
   b. Encephalopathy with cranial nerve palsies and convulsions
   c. Vertigo, deafness and tinnitus
3. Ocular features
   a. Granulomatous anterior uveitis

    b. Multiple uneven elevated cloudy patches coalescing to form bilateral exudative retinal detachments
    c. Vitritis
    d. Macular oedema
    e. Disc hyperaemia

Sympathetic ophthalmia

Usually occurs in fellow eye following penetrating trauma. May also occur after cataract extraction and perforating corneal ulcers. May occur between 10 days and 50 years after injury

1. Symptoms
    a. Photophobia
    b. Red eye
    c. Blurring of vision
2. Signs
    a. Ciliary flush
    b. Koeppe nodules on iris
    c. Posterior synechiae
    d. Large mutton fat keratic precipitates
    e. Retinal oedema
    f. Yellow white spots in retina (Dalen-Fuchs nodules)
    g. Swollen optic disc
3. Histology
    a. Panuveal cellular infiltration
    b. Pale islands of epithelioid macrophages and giant cells among hyperchromatic infiltrating lymphocytes
    c. Phagocytosed melanin in the cytoplasm of epithelioid and giant cells
    d. Dalen-Fuchs nodules. Nodules of ciliary epithelial cells and epithelioid macrophages beneath and between the pigmented and nonpigmented layers of the ciliary epithelium. These nodules are also found in ocular tuberculosis and Vogt-Koyanagi-Harada syndrome

Bird shot retinochoroidopathy

Affects patients over the age of 40. Increased incidence of HLA-A29. Females > Males
Ocular features
    a. Usually bilateral
    b. Mild anterior chamber activity
    c. Vitritis
    d. Chorioretinal lesions, depigmented spots at the level of the retinal pigment epithelium
    e. Retinal vasculitis
    f. Cystoid macular oedema
    g. Optic disc swelling

Acute multifocal placoid pigment epitheliopathy (AMPPE)
Affects young adults. 'Flu-like' prodromal syndrome may occur
1. Systemic features
   a. Thyroiditis
   b. Erythema nodosum
   c. Cerebral vasculitis
   d. Regional enteritis
2. Ocular features
   a. Usually affects both eyes
   b. Episcleritis
   c. Anterior uveitis
   d. Vitritis
   e. Cream coloured areas which coalesce in the posterior pole of one eye
   f. Vascular sheathing and disc oedema may occur

Serpiginous choroidopathy
Affects patients between 40 and 60 years of age
Ocular features
   a. Usually bilateral but asymmetrical
   b. Mild anterior uveitis
   c. Vitritis
   d. Cream coloured chorioretinal lesions (at RPE level) with hazy borders starting around the optic disc. Recurrent attacks with spread of the lesions
   e. Subretinal neovascularization may occur

Bilateral acute retinal necrosis (BARN)
Usually affects young patients
Ocular features
   a. Presents with acute visual loss
   b. Mild anterior uveitis
   c. Rubeosis may occur later
   d. Vitritis
   e. Necrosis of the retina beginning at the periphery and spreading inwards
   f. May lead to severe vitreous traction and retinal detachment

HLA association in uveitis
1. Ankylosing spondylitis — HLA-B27
2. Reiter's syndrome — HLA- B27
3. Behçet's syndrome — HLA-B5 (Japanese)
4. Vogt-Koyanagi-Harada syndrome — HLA-B22, BW54, DR4MT3
5. Sympathetic ophthalmitis — HLA-A11
6. Bird shot retinochoroidopathy — HLA-A29
7. Presumed ocular histoplasmosis — HLA-B7

Management of uveitis
Exact management will depend on type of uveitis
1. Exclude and treat any underlying cause, e.g. syphilitic uveitis
2. Exclude and treat complications, e.g. glaucoma
3. Steroids
   a. Topical
   b. Subconjunctival
   c. Retrobulbar
   d. Systemic
4. Mydriatics
   a. Prevent synechiae
   b. Reduce ciliary spasm
   c. Reduce vascular permeability, particularly atropine
5. Immunosuppressives, e.g. azathioprine

ENDOPHTHALMITIS

Inflammation of one or more coats of the eye and
adjacent intraocular spaces. Clinically used to describe potentially
destructive inflammation in the retina, choroid and adjacent
intraocular spaces

Types
1. Infectious
   a. Exogenous, e.g. secondary to intraocular surgery
   b. Endogenous, e.g. secondary to bacterial carditis
2. Non-infectious
   a. Lens induced
   b. Foreign bodies, e.g. copper and ophthalmia nodosa from
      caterpillar hairs

Symptoms
1. Pain
2. Decreased visual acuity
3. Ocular discharge
4. Headache
5. Red eye
6. Photophobia

Signs
1. Eyelid swelling
2. Red eye
3. Conjunctival oedema (chemosis)
4. Increase in white cells in anterior chamber
5. Fibrin in anterior chamber
6. Hypopyon
7. Retrolenticular cells
8. Decreased red reflex

9. Retinal haemorrhages or 'puff-balls' in the vitreous cavity
10. Vitreous clouding (may be masked if vitrectomy and gas or silicone oil have been injected into eye)

Causes of postoperative endophthalmitis
1. Gram Positive bacteria (90%)
   a. *Staph. epidermidis* (20–50%) ⎫
   b. *Staph. aureus*
   c. *Strep. pneumoniae*
   d. *Strep. viridans*   ⎬ aerobic
   e. *Strep. pyogenes*
   f. Corynebacterium   ⎭
   g. Peptostreptococcus   ⎫
   h. *Propionibacterium acnes* ⎬ anaerobic
   i. Clostridium   ⎭
2. Gram negative bacteria (7%)
   a. *Pseudomonas aeruginosa*
   b. Proteus
   c. *Haemophilus influenzae*
   d. *Klebsiella pneumoniae*
   e. *Escherichia coli*
   f. *Enterobacter aerogenes*
3. Fungi (3%)
   Present later (one or more weeks)
   a. Aspergillus
   b. Candida
   c. Cephalosporium
   d. Paecilomyces
   e. Penicillium

Commonest infecting organisms after filtering bleb surgery
1. Streptococci (57%)
2. *Haemophilus influenzae* (23%)
3. *Staph. aureus*

Causes of endogenous endophthalmitis
1. Fungal
   a. *Candida albicans* (75–80% of all endogenous endophthalmitis)
   b. *Aspergillus*
2. Bacterial
   a. *Neisseria meningitidis*
   b. *Streptococcus*
   c. *Staph. aureus*
   d. *Bacillus cereus*
   e. *Nocardia asteroides*
3. Viral, e.g. cytomegalovirus infection in AIDS. However, usually posterior uveitis rather than endophthalmitis

Management of endophthalmitis
Exact details depend on type and circumstances of endophthalmitis
1. Diagnosis
   a. Clinical features
   b. Lid swabs
   c. Anterior chamber/vitreous tap
      Gram and Giemsa stain
      Centrifuge vitreous to concentrate organisms and filter
      Blood agar ⎤
      Chocolate agar ⎥
      Cooked meat broth ⎬ media
      Sabouraud's ⎦
      Liaise with microbiologist
   d. Systemic cultures if associated primary or secondary
      septicaemia
2. Treatment
   a. Antibiotics
      (i) Topical (intensive and high concentration)
      (ii) Subconjunctival
      (iii) Intraocular — low volume, exact dose, no preservatives
      (iv) Systemic
   b. Vitrectomy
   c. Steroids
      (i) Topical
      (ii) Systemic

The glaucomas

Definition
A group of conditions characterized by optic disc cupping and field loss, in which the intraocular pressure is sufficiently raised to impair normal function of the optic nerve

THE CILIARY BODY

1. Anatomy
   a. Triangular in cross section, extending from ora serrata to scleral spur. 6 mm in width
   b. Anterior surface — shortest. Uveal portion of the trabecular meshwork
   c. Outer surface — lies against sclera. Lines potential suprachoroidal space
   d. Inner surface. Posterior $\frac{2}{3}$ is the pars plana. Anterior $\frac{1}{3}$ is the pars plicata. Pars plicata has 70 ciliary processes 0.8 mm high, 1 mm wide
2. Histology
   a. Uveal portion
      (i) Ciliary muscle (unstriated)
      (ii) Layer of vessels from major circle of iris (ciliary loops)
      (iii) Basal lamina continuous with Bruch's membrane
   b. Epithelial portion
      (i) Inner nonpigmented epithelium portion equivalent to sensory retina. Basal lamina continuous with internal limiting membrane of retina
      (ii) Outer pigmented epithelium equivalent to retinal pigment epithelium. Zonula occludens present. Basal lamina continuous with cuticular layer of Bruch's membrane
3. Blood supply — major circle of iris from 2 long ciliary arteries and 7 anterior ciliary arteries
4. Nerve supply
   a. Ciliary muscle — post-ganglionic parasympathetic fibres from oculomotor nerve via short ciliary nerves

  b. Blood vessels — sympathetic fibres also via short ciliary
     nerves
5. Functions
   a. Aqueous humour formation
      (i) Ultrafiltration
      (ii) Active secretion
   b. Accommodation
   c. Control of aqueous outflow
   d. Secretion of hyaluronic acid into the vitreous
   e. Blood aqueous barrier
6. Embryology
   a. Formed by fusion of optic cup (neuroectoderm) and
      surrounding mesoderm
   b. Ciliary processes formed from epithelium of developing
      retina
   c. Ciliary muscle formed from mesoderm — longitudinal fibres
      formed by 4 months; circular fibres formed by 6 months
   d. Aqueous circulation starts at 6 or 7 months

TRABECULAR MESHWORK

Encircles the circumference of the anterior chamber
1. Uveal meshwork — cord-shaped collagenous core surrounded
   by endothelial cells. Openings up to 70 μm in diameter. Linked
   to ciliary muscle
2. Corneoscleral meshwork — sheet-like beams insert into scleral
   spur. Openings up to 30 μm in diameter
3. Juxtacanalicular tissue — links corneoscleral trabeculae with
   Schlemm's canal endothelium. Trabecular organization absent.
   Openings 4–7 μm in width

CANAL OF SCHLEMM

1. Oval channel encircling circumference of the anterior chamber
2. Inner surface is in contact with juxtacanalicular tissue
3. Outer surface buried in corneoscleral stroma
4. Lined with single layer of endothelial cells
5. Passage of aqueous from trabecular meshwork to canal is
   controversial.
   Possibilities:
   a. Leaky endothelial cell junctions
   b. Transcellular channels
   c. Giant vacuoles (pinocytosis)
6. Canal connected to the venous system by 25–35 collector
   channels

AQUEOUS DRAINAGE

1. Conventional route — intraocular pressure dependent. Drains to Schlemm's canal, then deep scleral plexus into anterior ciliary and episcleral veins or into conjunctival aqueous veins
2. Uveoscleral route — intraocular pressure independent. Drains via anterior ciliary body face to suprachoroidal space, then to uveal or vortex veins or trans-sclerally to orbital veins

FEATURES OF THE ANTERIOR CHAMBER ANGLE (ON GONIOSCOPY)

1. Schwalbe's line — seen anteriorly. Peripheral termination of Descemet's membrane. Prominent and anterior in 15% of normal eyes (posterior embryotoxon)
2. Trabecular meshwork — from Schwalbe's line to scleral spur. More pigmented posteriorly
3. Schlemm's canal — sometimes seen behind posterior trabecular meshwork especially if filled with blood
4. Scleral spur — most anterior part of sclera. Site of attachment of longitudinal bundle of ciliary muscle
5. Ciliary body — brown band just behind scleral spur
6. Peripheral iris
7. Iris processes — insert from iris to scleral spur. More prominent in childhood
8. Iris blood vessels — circular are commonest. Radial are rarer

Angle width grading
Grade 4 — widest angle opening (35–45°)
    — ciliary body easily seen
    — seen in high myopia and aphakia
    — closure impossible
Grade 3 — scleral spur visible
    — closure impossible
Grade 2 — trabecular meshwork seen
    — angle closure possible but unlikely
Grade 1 — Schwalbe's line and top of trabecular meshwork seen
    — high risk of angle closure
Grade 0 — iridocorneal contact
    — complete closed angle

Abnormal gonioscopic findings
1. Blood in Schlemm's canal
   a. Secondary to gonioscopy
   b. Carotid-cavernous fistula
   c. Superior vena cava obstruction
   d. Sturge-Weber syndrome
   e. Ocular hypotony

2. Abnormal angle blood vessels
   a. Neovascular glaucoma
   b. Anterior uveitis
   c. Fuchs' heterochromic cyclitis
3. Hyperpigmented angle
   a. Pigment dispersion syndrome
   b. Pseudoexfoliation syndrome
   c. Laser iridotomy
   d. Anterior segment surgery
   e. Longstanding iritis
   f. Trauma
   g. Melanoma
   h. Increasing age
4. Peripheral anterior synechiae
   a. Angle closure
   b. Uveitis
   c. Neovascularization
   d. Loss of anterior chamber
   e. Iris bombé
   f. Essential iris atrophy
   g. Tumour of ciliary body
   h. Cleavage syndromes

AQUEOUS HUMOUR

1. Fills anterior and posterior chamber
2. Volume of anterior chamber aqueous — 0.25 ml
3. Volume of posterior chamber aqueous — 0.06 ml
4. Refractive index — 1.336
5. Production rate — 2–3 μl/min
6. Drainage rate. — 2 μl/min (conventional route)
   — 0.2 μl/min (uveoscleral route)
7. Composition varies between posterior and anterior chambers
   $\left.\begin{array}{l} [Na^+] \\ {[Cl^-]} \end{array}\right\}$ lower in posterior chamber
   $\left.\begin{array}{l} [PO_4^-] \\ {[HCO_3^-]} \end{array}\right\}$ higher in posterior chamber

INTRAOCULAR PRESSURE

1. Dependent on balance between inflow and outflow of aqueous humour
2. Normally 10–22 mmHg greater than atmospheric pressure
3. Variation of 1–2 mmHg with heartbeat and respiration
4. Diurnal variation of 2–3 mmHg. Highest on awakening, lowest during evening
5. Increases transiently on lying down and Valsalva manoeuvre

Measurement of intraocular pressure
1. Indentation tonometry. Plunger indents a soft eye more than a hard eye
   a. Schiotz tonometer. Scleral rigidity affects accuracy of measurement — underestimation if rigidity low, e.g. myopia, dysthyroid disease, miotic treatment
   b. Pneumotonometer. Detects change of gas flow through a flexible diaphragm
2. Applanation tonometry. Relies on application of Imbert-Fick principle (the force required to flatten an area of a sphere is proportional to the pressure within the sphere)
   a. Goldmann's tonometer. When the flattened area is 3.06 mm the surface tension of tears balances the elastic force of the cornea. Grams force × 10 is directly convertible into mmHg
   b. MacKay-Marg tonometer. Partly applanation, partly indentation. 1.5 mm plunger protruding 5 μm beyond surface footplate. Can be used on scarred, irregular corneas
   c. Non-contact tonometer. Uses an air puff to flatten cornea. Light reflected from flattened corneal surface to photo-receptor. Tends to overestimate intraocular pressure especially in higher ranges

CHRONIC OPEN ANGLE GLAUCOMA

Affects 0.5–1.0% of population over 40 years of age
Is responsible for 20% of blind registrations in the UK
1. Pathogenesis
   Histological features include:
   a. Trabecular meshwork
      (i) Endothelial cell loss
      (ii) Alterations to extracellular matrix
      (iii) Loss of giant vacuoles from canal of Schlemm
      (iv) Increase in trabecular thickness
      (v) Excessive fusion of trabeculae
      (vi) Hyperpigmentation of meshwork cells
   b. Optic disc
      (i) Compression and collapse of lamina cribrosa collagen bundles
      (ii) Swollen axons at optic nerve head with hold up of axoplasmic transport
      (iii) Eventual selective axonal destruction in 'hour glass' pattern at optic disc
   Changes in the trabecular meshwork may impede aqueous outflow, and thus increase intraocular pressure
   Visual loss may occur by
   a. Direct mechanical effects on nerve fibres
   b. Vascular insufficiency to optic nerve head
   Characteristic pattern of nerve loss may relate to regional

differences in axonal support, lamina cribrosa or vascular
supply to optic nerve head
2. Criteria for diagnosis
   a. Intraocular pressure > 21 mmHg
   b. Open angle on gonioscopy
   c. Glaucomatous cupping of the optic disc
   d. Glaucomatous visual field defect
3. Optic disc changes
   a. Cup/disc ratio
      (i) Normal < 0.3 (increases with age)
      (ii) Asymmetry of > 0.2 is suspicious
      (iii) Notching of rim is suspicious
   b. Pallor
      (i) Area of disc lacking small vessels
      (ii) Does not increase with age
   c. Nasal shift of blood vessels at the disc
   d. Haemorrhages on the disc or disc margin
   e. Retinal nerve fibre layer atrophy — visible in red-free light
   f. Difficulties arise in
      (i) high myopia
      (ii) congenital disc anomalies
      (iii) media opacities
      (iv) small pupils
4. Visual field
   a. Paracentral scotoma 10–20° from the blind spot
   b. Arcuate scotoma (Seidel's scotoma)
   c. Arcuate scotoma with breakthrough to the periphery
   d. Nasal step (Roenne scotoma)
   e. Temporal wedge
   f. Generalized constriction often with residual island
5. Visual field testing
   a. Kinetic
      (i) Bjerrum's screen (central 30° only)
      (ii) Lister perimeter (peripheral fields only)
      (iii) Goldmann perimeter (evaluates whole field
   b. Static
      (i) Adapted Goldmann perimeter
      (ii) Friedmann perimeter
      (iii) Computer assisted — automatically tests
           suprathreshold and threshold stimuli and quantifies
           depth of field defect
6. Associations
   a. Ocular
      (i) High myopia
      (ii) Retinal vein occlusion
      (iii) Retinal detachment
      (iv) Fuch's endothelial dystrophy
      (v) Retinitis pigmentosa
   b. Systemic — diabetes mellitus

Treatment of chronic open angle glaucoma
1. Medical
   a. Topical
      (i) Beta-blockers
      (ii) Miotics
      (iii) Sympathomimetics
   b. Systemic — carbonic anhydrase inhibitors
2. Surgical
   a. Argon laser trabeculoplasty
   b. Trabeculectomy
   c. Drainage tube
   d. Destruction of ciliary processes

Argon laser trabeculoplasty
1. Indications
   a. Visual field loss continuing on maximum tolerated medical
      therapy
   b. High intraocular pressure uncontrolled by medications
   c. Poor compliance of medical therapy
   d. Replacement of poorly tolerated medication
   e. Poor response to glaucoma surgery
   f. Medically unfit for glaucoma surgery
2. Good response
   a. Chronic open angle glaucoma
   b. Pseudoexfoliative glaucoma
   c. Pigmentary glaucoma
3. Variable response
   a. Aphakic open angle glaucoma
   b. Angle recession glaucoma
4. Poor response
   a. Steroid induced glaucoma
   b. Ghost cell glaucoma
   c. Uveitic glaucoma
   d. Juvenile open angle glaucoma
   e. Iridocorneal endothelial syndrome
   f. Iridocorneal mesodermal dysgenesis
   g. Glaucoma due to elevated episcleral venous pressure
5. Complications
   a. Transient rise of intraocular pressure
   b. Persistent rise of intraocular pressure
   c. Transient blurring of vision
   d. Worsening of visual field defects
   e. Anterior uveitis
   f. Peripheral anterior synechiae

Trabeculectomy
1. Indications
   a. Continuing visual field loss on maximum tolerated medical
      therapy

   b. High intraocular pressure uncontrolled by medications
   c. Poor compliance of medical therapy
   d. Poor response after argon laser trabeculoplasty
2. Poor response
   a. Coloured patients
   b. Glaucoma due to elevated episcleral venous pressure
3. Complications
   a. Flat anterior chamber
   b. Hypotony
   c. Choroidal detachments and folds
   d. Hyphaema
   e. Malignant (ciliary block) glaucoma
   f. Cataract formation (10%)
   g. Visual field deterioration
   h. Endophthalmitis (early or late)

OCULAR HYPERTENSION

High intraocular pressure with normal optic discs and visual fields
Consider treatment if
1. Fellow eye has disc and field changes
2. Intraocular pressure > 30 mmHg
3. Rising intraocular pressure
4. Family history of glaucoma
5. Diabetic patient
6. > 70 years old
7. Only eye
8. Optic disc splinter haemorrhage

LOW TENSION GLAUCOMA

Normal intraocular pressure associated with increasing optic disc
cupping and visual field loss
1. Pathogenesis
   a. Unknown
   b. May be related to poor optic nerve head perfusion
   c. Important to exclude transient rises in intraocular pressure
     and also cranial space occupying lesions, e.g. meningioma
2. Prognosis is poor

ACUTE ANGLE CLOSURE GLAUCOMA

1. Incidence
   a. 1 in 1000 people over 40 years
   b. Male to female ratio is 1:4
2. Symptoms
   a. Pain
   b. Coloured haloes
   c. Headache

    d. Nausea, vomiting
    e. Previous history of subacute attacks
3. Signs
    a. Reduced vision
    b. Ciliary injection
    c. Corneal oedema
    d. Mid-dilated, vertically oval pupil
    e. Shallow anterior chamber
    f. Flare and cells in anterior chamber
    g. Congested iris vessels
    h. Iris stromal oedema
    i. Central retinal artery pulsation
4. Predisposing factors
    a. Hypermetropia
    b. Small corneal diameter
    c. Short axial length of globe
    d. Large crystalline lens
    e. Shallow anterior chamber (< 2.5 mm)
5. Provocative tests
    Used in latent or subacute cases. Positive result if 8 mmHg pressure rise occurs in one hour.
    Types
    a. Physiological
       (i) Dark room test
      (ii) Prone test
     (iii) Prone dark room test (patient must remain awake)
    b. Pharmacological
       (i) 10% phenylephrine (reversible with thymoxamine)
      (ii) 10% phenylephrine and 2% pilocarpine
6. Sequelae
    a. Poor vision
    b. Sectorial iris atrophy
    c. Spiralling of iris fibres
    d. Iris hole (pseudopolycoria)
    e. Large irregular pupil
    f. Glaukomflecken
    g. Peripheral anterior synechiae
    h. Chronic corneal oedema
7. Treatment
    a. Initial
       (i) Acetazolamide 500 mg i.v., then 250 mg four times a day orally
      (ii) Pilocarpine 4% every 15 min for one hour, then four times a day
     (iii) Topical steroids
     (iv) Osmotic agents, e.g. glycerol 1–2 g/kg body weight orally in lemon juice and/or mannitol 1–2 g/kg body weight (20% solution) given i.v. over 30 min

Side effects of osmotic agents — headache
— backache
— vertigo
— nausea
— mental confusion
— cardiovascular
overload
— pulmonary oedema
— diabetes (with
glycerol)
b. Late
(i) Medical therapy if infirm
(ii) Surgery — peripheral iridectomy
— laser iridotomy
— filtration surgery
— iridectomy/iridotomy on fellow eye

CHRONIC CLOSED ANGLE GLAUCOMA

1. Clinical features
   a. Painless
   b. Angle partially closed
   c. Peripheral anterior synechiae
   d. Intraocular pressure mildly elevated
   e. Visual field defects
2. Treatment — depends on degree of peripheral anterior synechiae
   a. Medical
   b. Surgical — peripheral iridotomy
   — laser iridotomy
   — filtration surgery

SECONDARY OPEN ANGLE GLAUCOMA

1. Pretrabecular. Membrane preventing access to angle
   a. Fibrovascular membrane (neovascularization)
   b. Endothelial membrane (iridocorneal endothelial syndrome)
      (i) Cogan Reese (iris naevus)
      (ii) Chandler
      (iii) Essential iris atrophy
   c. Epithelial downgrowth
   d. Fibrous ingrowth
2. Trabecular
   a. Clogging of meshwork
      (i) Red blood cells — hyphaema
      — ghost cell glaucoma

(ii) Macrophages — haemolytic
— phacoanaphylactic
— melanomalytic
(iii) Neoplastic cells — malignant tumours
— neurofibromatosis
— juvenile xanthogranuloma
(iv) Pigment — pigmentary glaucoma
— pseudoexfoliation
— longstanding uveitis
— malignant melanoma
(v) Protein — uveitis— lens induced
(vi) Alpha-chymotrypsin induced
(vii) Vitreous disruption
(viii) Pseudoexfoliative material
b. Alteration of meshwork
(i) Oedema — uveitis
— scleritis
— alkali burns
(ii) Trauma — angle recession
(iii) Intraocular foreign body — haemosiderosis and
chalcosis
(iv) Steroid induced
3. Post trabecular. High episcleral venous pressure preventing outflow.
a. Carotid-cavernous fistula
b. Cavernous sinus thrombosis
c. Orbital tumours
d. Dysthyroid eye disease
e. Superior vena cava obstruction
f. Mediastinal tumours
g. Sturge-Weber syndrome
h. Idiopathic

SECONDARY CLOSED ANGLE GLAUCOMA
1. With pupil block
a. Intumescent lens
b. Subluxation of lens
c. Following lens extraction
d. Pseudophakia, especially intracapsular lens extraction and anterior chamber implant
e. Iris bombé due to ring synechiae
2. Without pupil block
a. Malignant (ciliary block) glaucoma *Bymydriatic!! → vitrecto or PoJ vij*
b. Following scleral buckling
c. Following panretinal photocoagulation
d. Intraocular tumours→ *mm, mets, Lymph, leuh; RB, (×6)*
e. Cysts of iris and ciliary body
Downgrowth.

   f. Retrolental tissue contraction
     (i) Retinopathy of prematurity
     (ii) Persistent hyperplastic primary vitreous

Lens induced glaucomas
1. Phakomorphic — causes pupil block and secondary angle closure by
   a. Lens intumescence
   b. Lens dislocation (anteriorly and posteriorly)
2. Phacolytic — leak of lens proteins. Clogs trabecular meshwork
3. Phacoanaphylactic — sensitization of eye or its fellow to lens protein. Inflammatory material clogs trabecular meshwork

Pseudoexfoliation syndrome   *⊖ Steroid resp.*
1. Presence of widely dispersed abnormal amyloid-like deposits
2. Commoner in Scandinavians
3. Bilateral asymmetrical condition often more advanced in one eye
4. 70% associated with raised intraocular pressure
5. Features
   a. Flakes of material seen on
      (i)   anterior lens capsule
      (ii) pupil margin
      (iii) ciliary processes
      (iv) zonule
      (v)   anterior hyaloid face
   b. Pigmented trabecular meshwork
   c. Pigment on Schwalbe's line (Sampoelesi's line)
6. Treatment of glaucoma is difficult *⊕ ALT OK*

Pigment dispersion syndrome   *⊖ steroid resp.*
1. Bilateral disorder
2. Often affects myopic young men
3. Probably due to iris trauma from zonules
4. Features
   a. Radial iris transillumination in mid-periphery
   b. Pigment loss from posterior iris pigment epithelium
   c. Pigment deposited on
      (i)   Corneal endothelium (Krukenberg spindle)
      (ii) Trabecular meshwork
      (iii) Schwalbe's line (Sampoelesi's line)
      (iv) Lens
      (v)   Zonule
      (vi) Iris
5. May be associated with open angle glaucoma
6. Treatment of glaucoma difficult
   ✓ ALT is good.

NEOVASCULAR GLAUCOMA

Presence of glaucoma with a fibrovascular membrane occluding the drainage angle
1. Pathogenesis
    a. Stimulus to new vessel formation usually related to posterior segment ischaemia
    b. Proliferation begins at pupil margin and spreads centrifugally
    c. Progressive peripheral anterior synechiae result in angle closure
2. Causes
    a. Vascular
        (i) Retinal vein occlusion
        (ii) Diabetic retinopathy
        (iii) Retinal artery occlusion
        (iv) Carotid artery occlusive disease
    b. Inflammatory
        (i) Chronic uveitis
        (ii) Endophthalmitis
        (iii) Sympathetic ophthalmia
        (iv) Longstanding retinal detachment
    c. Neoplastic
        (i) Retinoblastoma
        (ii) Choroidal malignant melanoma
        (iii) Choroidal metastases
    d. Surgical
        (i) Cataract extraction
        (ii) Vitrectomy
        (iii) Retinal detachment surgery
3. Treatment
    a. Removal of stimulus, e.g. retinal panphotocoagulation
    b. Cyclocryotherapy
    c. Glaucoma implants, e.g. Molteno tube
    d. Palliation
        (i) Topical atropine and steroids
        (ii) Retrobulbar alcohol
        (iii) Enucleation

PRIMARY CONGENITAL GLAUCOMA

1. Autosomal recessive
2. Affects 1 in 10 000 live births
3. Males > Females (3:1)
4. May be manifest at birth or develop later
5. Features
    a. Lacrimation
    b. Photophobia
    c. Eye rubbing

    d. Buphthalmos (with early onset)
       (i) Corneal diameter < 13 mm
       (ii) Corneal oedema
       (iii) 'Healed' splits in Descemet's membrane (Haab's striae)
    e. Myopia
    f. Variable optic disc cupping
 6. Gonioscopic findings
    a. Barkan's membrane
    b. Thickening of trabecular sheets
    c. Insertion of iris above scleral spur
    d. Peripheral iris stroma hypoplasia
 7. Treatment
    a. Goniotomy
    b. Trabeculotomy
    c. Trabeculectomy

S – sclerocornea
T – Trauma – forceps
U – UP IOP !! Glaucoma.
M – mucopolysacch.
P – Peters anomaly.
E – Endothelial dyst (CHED)
D – Dermoid.

Differential diagnosis of cloudy cornea at birth
 1. Glaucoma, primary or secondary *Key!*
 2. Trauma *– forceps –*
 3. Rubella and other intrauterine infections *TORCHS.*
 4. Mucopolysaccharidoses *all exapt Hunter & sanfilipo*
 5. Mucolipidoses
 6. Peter's anomaly
    Dermoid.

SECONDARY CONGENITAL GLAUCOMA

Causes (and % with glaucoma)
 1. Rubella (10%)
 2. Aniridia (50%)
 3. Microcornea (60% closed angle)
 4. Neurofibromatosis (25%)
 5. Sturge-Weber syndrome (50%)
 6. Mesodermal dysgenesis syndromes (50%)
 7. Lowe's syndrome (50%)

Aniridia (sporadic or autosomal dominant)
Features
    a. Poor vision *hypoplastic macula*
    b. Nystagmus
    c. Photophobia
    d. Complete or partial absence of iris
    e. Angle anomalies
    f. Glaucoma — 50%
    g. Corneal pannus
    h. Epibulbar dermoids
    i. Cataract
    j. Lens subluxation
    k. Hypoplastic macula *– ↓ VA –*

l. Hypoplastic optic disc
m. Wilms' tumour in 20% of sporadic cases

Mesodermal dysgenesis
1. Axenfeld's anomaly
   Features
   a. Posterior embryotoxon
   b. Iris strands to Schwalbe's line
   c. Not associated with glaucoma
2. Reiger's syndrome (autosomal dominant)
   Features
   a. Abnormal dentition
   b. Maxillary hypoplasia
   c. Bilateral ocular involvement
       (i) Posterior embryotoxon
       (ii) Iris strands
       (iii) Peripheral anterior synechiae
       (iv) Pupillary distortion
       (v) Peripheral corneal opacification
       (vi) Ectropion uveae
       (vii) Glaucoma in 50% of cases
3. Peter's anomaly (AUT recessive)
   a. 80% bilateral
   b. Associated with central defect of Descemet's membrane
   c. Types
       (i) Central posterior corneal stromal opacity
       (ii) Posterior stromal opacity with iris adhesions
       (iii) Posterior corneal defect with lens adhesions
   d. Glaucoma in 50% of cases

Lens

MACROSCOPIC ANATOMY

1. Biconvex, transparent
2. Diameter 10 mm
3. Thickness 4 mm
4. Anterior face radius 10 mm
5. Posterior face radius 6 mm

RELATIONS OF THE LENS

1. Anteriorly — iris and pupil
2. Posteriorly — patella fossa of anterior vitreous face
3. Surround — lens equator 0.5 mm from ciliary body

MICROSCOPIC ANATOMY

1. Lens capsule
   a. Basement membrane of lens epithelium
   b. Smooth, acellular, elastic
   c. Composed of collagen and acid mucopolysaccharides
   d. Thickest distal to zonule insertion
2. Lens zonule (of Zinn)
   a. Suspensory ligament of lens
   b. Composed of fine collagen fibrils
   c. Origin — from pigmented layer of ciliary body epithelium, from sides of processes and valleys. Extends to pars plana
   d. Insertion — posterior fibres insert anteriorly 1 mm below equator. Anterior fibres insert posteriorly 0.5 mm below equator. These two groups are separated by Petit's canal. Form fine indentations in lens surface
3. Anterior lens epithelium — single cuboidal layer epithelium
4. Lens fibres
   a. Roughly hexagonal in cross section
   b. 2100–2300 fibres; each fibre is a single cell
   c. Dimensions
      (i) 8–12 μm long

        (ii) 7 μm wide in cortical zone, 5 μm in nuclear zone and
            2 μm near sutures
  d. Produced throughout life
  e. Cell division at lens equator
  f. Fibres elongate but initially have contact with epithelium
     and lens capsule
  g. Nuclei predominantly in equatorial zone
  h. Fibres shed towards lens centre
  i. Parallel to curved lens surface
  j. Radially placed
  k. Relatively few organelles, small nuclei
  l. Intercellular substance joining cells at sutures
  m. Fetal suture
     (i) anteriorly 'Y' shaped
     (ii) posteriorly 'λ' shaped
  n. Post fetal sutures increasingly complex
  o. Old fibres
     (i) Compressed centrally and lose nuclei
     (ii) Form lens nucleus
5. Lens zone — concentric areas of differing refractive index
  a. Subcapsular zone — clear
  b. Cortical zone — newly formed fibres
  c. Nuclear zone — old dense central fibres
     (i) Embryonic
     (ii) Fetal
     (iii) Infantile
     (iv) Adult

EMBRYOLOGY

1. 3 week stage — lens placode from surface ectoderm
2. 6 week stage — lens vesicle. Further development requiring
   normal neuroretina in appropriate position
3. 12 week stage — tunica vasculosa lentis
4. 28–38 week stage — degeneration of tunica vasculosa lentis

PHYSIOLOGY

1. Function — refraction of light to produce clear retinal image
   (= 35% of refracting power of eye)
2. Growth
  a. New fibres formed throughout life
  b. Weight at birth: 100 mg
  c. Weight at 65 years: 250 mg
  d. Width and cell density increases with age
  e. Radius of surfaces decreases with age
3. Transparency
  a. 80% of light between 400 nm and 1400 nm transmitted

b. Related to
   (i) Scarcity of cellular organelles
   (ii) Little extracellular space
   (iii) High proportion of soluble proteins
c. Refractive index variable
   (i) Cortex: 1.38
   (ii) Nucleus: 1.40
d. Ageing
   (i) Yellowing of nucleus
   (ii) Increased absorption of ultraviolet light aiding retinal protection
   (iii) Fluorescent compounds produced (chromatophores)
4. Metabolism
   a. Anaerobic
   b. 85% of glucose by glycolysis
   c. Lactate diffuses into aqueous
   d. 15% by pentose phosphate shunt
   e. Highest metabolic rate in cortex
   f. Energy required for
      (i) Glutathione production
      (ii) Large molecule production
      (iii) Ion transportation
5. Composition
   a. 64% water
   b. 35% protein (highest in body tissue)
   c. 1% lipid, trace elements, carbohydrates
   d. Proteins
      (i) Insoluble albuminoid 12%
      (ii) α crystallins 31%
      (iii) β heavy crystallins ⎫ 55%
      (iv) β light crystallins ⎭
      (v) γ crystallins 2%
   e. [K] lens : × 25 [K] aqueous
   f. [Na] lens : × 0.1 [Na] aqueous
   g. [Amino acid] lens : ×6 [amino acid] aqueous
   h. High glutathione content maintains reduced proteins and membrane pump integrity
6. Accommodation
   a. Lens essentially noncompressible
   b. Resting state — globular
   c. Relaxed ciliary ring tightens zonules and produces a flattened lens
   d. Ciliary contraction relaxes zonules and results in an increasingly spherical lens. Anterior surface shows most increase in curvature
   e. Ageing
      (i) Less deformable lens
      (ii) Reduced accommodation
      (iii) Presbyopia

DISORDERS OF LENS SHAPE AND POSITION

1. Coloboma
   a. Congenital
   b. Absence of segment of zonule
   c. Lens rim relaxes
   d. Lower quadrants
   e. Associated with iris, choroidal and optic nerve colobomata and giant retinal tears
2. Lenticonus
   a. Conical shape relative to lens surface
   b. Anterior or posterior
   c. Oil drop sign on eliciting red reflex
   d. Irregular myopic lenticular astigmatism
   e. Anterior lenticonus associated with cataract and Alport's syndrome
       (i) Autosomal recessive
       (ii) Anterior lenticonus
       (iii) Endothelial changes
       (iv) Cataract
       (v) Spherophakia
       (vi) Deafness
       (vii) Nephritis
   f. Posterior lenticonus unilateral and associated with cataract
3. Lentiglobus — generalized hemispherical deformity
4. Microphakia
   a. Small lens due to arrested lens development
   b. Associated with Lowe's syndrome
5. Microspherophakia
   a. Small spherical lens, usually bilateral
   b. Zonule visible on pupillary dilatation
   c. Iridodonesis
   d. Zonular rupture common
   e. Pupil block glaucoma occurs → *helped by cycloplegia worsened by miotics.*
   f. Associations
       (i) Familial
       (ii) Weill-Marchesani syndrome
       (iii) Marfan's syndrome
       (iv) Hyperlysinaemia
6. Ectopia lentis
   a. Subluxation or dislocation of lens
   b. Results from zonular rupture
   c. Produces loss of accommodation
   d. Refractive errors may occur
       (i) Subluxation — myopia or astigmatism
       (ii) Dislocation — hypermetropia
   e. Glaucoma due to lens position or uveitis

Causes of a dislocated lens
1. Hereditary causes
   a. Marfan's syndrome
   b. Weill-Marchesani syndrome
   c. Homocystinuria
   d. Ehlers-Danlos syndrome
   e. Sulphite oxidase deficiency
   f. Hyperlysinaemia
   g. Familial ectopia lentis (autosomal recessive)
   h. Aniridia
2. Acquired causes
   a. Trauma — ocular contusion and couching
   b. Buphthalmos
   c. Anterior uveal tumours
   d. Syphilis
   e. Spontaneous (hypermature cataract)
   f. High myopia
   g. Chronic uveitis

Marfan's syndrome
Autosomal dominant. Mesodermal dysplasia
Possible defect of collagen cross linkages
Increased hydroxyproline and desmosine excretion
Clinical diagnosis — arm span > height
1. General features
   a. Dissecting aortic aneurysms
   b. Aortic regurgitation
   c. Arachnodactyly
   d. High arched palate
   e. Muscular underdevelopment
2. Ocular features
   a. Bilateral upward subluxation
   b. Nonprogressive subluxation, accommodation retained
   c. Microspherophakia
   d. Angle anomalies (glaucoma)
   e. Hypoplastic iris dilators
   f. Cornea plana and keratoconus
   g. Axial myopia
   h. Vitreoretinal degeneration and retinal detachment

Weill-Marchesani syndrome
Autosomal recessive. Disorder of connective tissue
1. General features
   a. Mental retardation
   b. Short stature
   c. Stubby fingers
   d. Joint stiffness

2. Ocular features
   a. Microphthalmos
   b. Myopia (−10 to −20 D)
   c. Microspherophakia
   d. Inferior, anterior or posterior dislocation of lens
   e. Glaucoma secondary to lens dislocation *→ R mydriatic*
   → bus extraction

Homocystinuria
Autosomal recessive. Deficiency of cystathionine synthetase
Variable activity produces variable clinical picture
Accumulation of methionine and homocysteine
Nitroprusside urine test and amino acid assays are diagnostic
1. General features
   a. Skeletal — osteoporosis, fractures
   b. CNS — mental retardation, seizures
   c. CVS — malar flush, thromboemboli (especially after general anaesthetic)
2. Ocular features
   a. Acquired zonular damage
   b. Downward subluxation
   c. Staphylomas
   d. Buphthalmos, myopia
   e. Glaucoma. Vitreoretinal degeneration
3. Treatment
   a. Vitamin B_6 (50% respond)
   b. Methionine-restricted diet
   c. Supplementary cysteine
   d. Folate

Ehlers–Danlos syndrome
Autosomal dominant, autosomal recessive or X-linked recessive
Major defect of type III collagen
At least nine types
1. General features
   a. Variable
   b. Hyperextensible joints
   c. Hyperextensible skin
   d. Easy bruising
   e. Poor wound healing
2. Ocular features
   a. Easy lid eversion (Metenier's sign)
   b. Epicanthic folds
   c. Myopia, microcornea
   d. Blue sclera
   e. Keratoconus
   f. Ectopia lentis
   g. Vitreous haemorrhage
   h. Angioid streaks
   i. Retinal detachment

Sulphite oxidase deficiency
Autosomal recessive
Possible deficiency of molybdenum
Increased urinary sulphite
1. General features
   a. Mental retardation
   b. Frontal bossing
2. Ocular features
   a. Enophthalmos
   b. Ectopia lentis
   c. Brushfield spots

Hyperlysinaemia
Autosomal recessive
Deficiency of lysine dehydrogenase
1. General features
   a. Motor ⎫
   b. Mental ⎬ retardation
   c. Growth ⎭
2. Ocular feature — microspherophakia

LENS INDUCED DISORDERS

1. Glaucoma
   a. Phacomorphic (due to lens shape)
   b. Phacolytic (due to capsular leakage)
   c. Lens displacement
2. Uveitis
   a. Phacoanaphylactic (autoimmune sensitivity to lens protein)
   b. Phacotoxic (toxic reaction to lens protein)

CATARACT

Definition
Any opacity within the lens. WHO estimates (1978) 15 million blind
(<3/60) from cataract (commonest cause of blindness)

Classification
1. According to age
   a. Congenital
   b. Infantile
   c. Juvenile
   d. Presenile
   e. Senile
2. According to stage
   a. Immature
   b. Stationary
   c. Progressive
   d. Mature

  e. Intumescent
  f. Hypermature (Morgagnian)
3. According to morphology
  a. Capsular
    (i) Congenital — anterior polar, pyramidal
    (ii) Acquired — infra red (glassblowers), mercury (grey), 'chlorpromazine' (white star)
  b. Subcapsular
    (i) Posterior — senile or secondary, e.g. dystrophia myotonica
    (ii) Anterior — glaucomflecken, Wilson's disease (green sunflower), miotic therapy
  c. Cortical
    (i) Congenital — blue/brown dot, coronary (supranuclear)
    (ii) Acquired — senile cuneiform
  d. Nuclear
    (i) Congenital — embryonal (cataracta centralis pulverulenta), lamellar with or without riders (genetic, metabolic and infective causes)
    (ii) Acquired — senile nuclear sclerosis
4. According to aetiology
  a. Not associated with ocular disease
  b. Associated with ocular disease
  c. Associated with systemic disease

Cataracts unassociated with ocular disease
Senile cataract (90% of > 70 year age group)
1. Type
  a. Anterior subcapsular due to fibrous metaplasia
  b. Posterior subcapsular due to epithelial cell migration
  c. Cortical
  d. Nuclear cataract is an exaggeration of ageing process
2. Risks
  a. Increased by
    (i) Smoking
    (ii) Dehydration, e.g. diarrhoea
    (iii) Ultraviolet light exposure
  b. Reduced by nonsteroidal anti-inflammatory drugs
3. Lens findings
  a. Increase in sodium ions, water (hydration), calcium ions, and insoluble proteins
  b. Reduction in potassium ions, amino acids and glutathione
  c. Changes in crystallins occur due to deamination, glycosylation, carbamylation, and sterol addition
  These changes result in
    (i) Protein unfolding
    (ii) Reduction in thiol groups
    (iii) Disulphide cross links

       (iv) Changes in surface charges (removal of positive
            charge)
       (v) Exposure of hydrophobic sites
      (vi) Protein aggregation
     (vii) Increased insoluble protein
    (viii) Reduced glutathione levels
4. Lens opacities occur due to
   a. Altered refractive index
   b. Large aggregates
   c. Differences of refractive index at interfaces

Cataracts associated with ocular disease
1. Congenital disorders
   a. Aniridia
   b. Hyperplastic primary vitreous
   c. Hereditary retinal disease
   d. Hereditary vitreoretinal disease
2. Acquired disorders
   a. Uveitis
   b. Glaucoma (glaucomflecken)
   c. Myopia
   d. Retinal detachment
   e. Neoplasia
   f. Drug treatment, e.g. steroids, miotics
   g. Trauma
       (i) Contusion (Vossius' ring)
      (ii) Rupture of lens
     (iii) Retained intraocular foreign body (siderosis, chalcosis)
     (iv) Electric shock
      (v) Radiation
     (vi) Alkali burns

Cataracts associated with systemic disease
1. Maternal infection
   a. Rubella
     15% of childbearing women susceptible
     Longlasting immunity follows infection
     Fetal risk 80% in first trimester
     General features
       (i) Stillbirth or abortion
      (ii) Deafness (90%)
     (iii) Cardiovascular defects, e.g. patent ductus arteriosus
     (iv) Intrauterine growth retardation
      (v) Psychomotor retardation
     (vi) Pneumonitis
     Ocular features
       (i) Occur in 30–60% of cases

    (ii) Cataract in 50%. Unilateral or bilateral. Nuclear or diffuse
   (iii) Viable virus in lens for 3 years
   (iv) Intense uveitis on lens extraction
    (v) Microphthalmos (15%)
   (vi) Retinopathy with 'salt and pepper' appearance
  (vii) Late disciform degeneration, therefore tendency to operate on unilateral cataracts in rubella
 (viii) Glaucoma (10%)
   (ix) Strabismus, nystagmus, refractive errors and optic atrophy

b. Cytomegalovirus inclusion disease
General features
    (i) Low birth weight
   (ii) Hepatosplenomegaly, jaundice
  (iii) Purpura, pneumonitis
  (iv) Cerebral calcification, deafness
   (v) Psychomotor retardation, seizures
Ocular features
    (i) Cataract
   (ii) Uveitis, microphthalmos
  (iii) Optic nerve hypoplasia, coloboma and atrophy
  (iv) Chorioretinitis

c. Toxoplasmosis
Infection of cats and spread via cats faeces
General features
Nervous system — convulsions
                 — mental retardation
                 — intracranial calcification
Ocular features — chorioretinal scars

2. Maternal drug ingestion
3. Maternal radiation
4. Chromosomal abnormalities, e.g. Down's syndrome (snowflake cataract)
5. Hereditary disorders, e.g. Marfan's syndrome and syndromes associated with retinitis pigmentosa
6. Cutaneous disorders
  a. Atopic dermatitis
     (i) Anterior or posterior stellate cataract
    (ii) Chronic keratoconjunctivitis
   (iii) Keratoconus
  b. Werner's syndrome (scleropoikiloderma)
  c. Schaefer's syndrome (congenital dyskeratoses)
  d. Rothmund's syndrome (infantile poikiloderma)
  e. Congenital ichthyosis
7. Systemic infections, e.g. syphilis
8. Systemic drugs, e.g. steroids, antimitotics and chlorpromazine

9. Metabolic disorders
   a. Diabetes mellitus (bilateral, white snowflake and may
      progress rapidly)
   b. Hypoglycaemic cataract
   c. Galactosaemia. Autosomal recessive. Impairment of
      galactose metabolism, excess reduced to dulcitol. Initially
      lens clear, osmotic cataract develops. 2 types of defect:
      (i) Galactose-1-phosphate uridyltransferase deficiency
          General features — onset in infancy with failure to thrive
                           — renal disease
                           — hepatosplenomegaly, cirrhosis
                           — anaemia, deafness
                           — mental retardation
                           — death unless milk and derivatives
                             removed from diet
      (ii) Galactokinase deficiency
           General features — systemically well
                            — Mild galactosaemia possibly
                              associated with presenile cataract
   d. Mannosidosis. Alpha-mannosidase deficiency
      General features
      'Hurler-like' syndrome (mental retardation, short stature,
      skeletal changes, hepatosplenomegaly)
      Ocular features
      (i) Posterior spoke-like capsular opacity
      (ii) No corneal changes unlike Hurler's syndrome
   e. Fabry's disease. Alpha-galactosidase A deficiency
      General features
      (i) Angiokeratomas
      (ii) Cardiovascular disorders
      (iii) Renal disorders
      (iv) Bouts of pain in digits
      Ocular features
      (i) Cornea verticillata
      (ii) Spoke-like cataract (25%)
   f. Lowe's syndrome. Defect of amino acid metabolism
      General features
      (i) Males > Females
      (ii) Mental retardation
      (iii) Renal dwarfism
      (iv) Osteomalacia
      (v) Muscular hypotonia
      (vi) Frontal prominence
      Ocular features
      (i) Congenital glaucoma (50%)
      (ii) Congenital cataract (100%)
      (iii) Small disc-like lens opacities in mother

g. Wilson's disease. Alpha-2-globulin (ceruloplasmin)
   deficiency
   General features.
      Hepatolenticular degeneration.
   Ocular features
      (i) Kayser Fleischer ring
      (ii) Green sunflower cataract
h. Hypocalcaemia due to hypoparathyroidism or
   pseudohypoparathyroidism (short stature and short 4th and
   5th metacarpals)
   Ocular features
      White dot or coloured crystal opacities
10. Muscular disorders.
    Dystrophia Myotonica. Autosomal dominant
    General features
    a. Wasting (temporalis, sternomastoid)
    b. Frontal balding
    c. Excessive contractility of muscles
    d. Hypogonadism
    e. Cardiac defects
    Ocular features
    a. Ptosis
    b. Christmas tree cataract (cortical polychromatic dusting)
    c. Light/near dissociation
    d. Pigmentary retinal changes

Assessment of a patient with cataract
1. History
   Variable and may include
   a. Changing refraction
   b. Increasing myopia (second sight)
   c. Gradually failing vision
   d. Worse vision whilst reading
   e. Worse vision in bright light
   f. Glare
   g. Ghosting (monocular diplopia)
   h. Monochromatic haloes
   i Past ocular disease
   j Past and present refractive status
2. Examination
   a. Vision (near, distance and with pinhole) also glare test
   b. Refraction
   c. Light projection
   d. Macular function tests
   e. Ocular adnexae
   f. Tears
   g. Cornea (scarring, pannus)
   h. Endothelium (guttata)
   i. Anterior chamber depth

j. Intraocular pressure
k. Pupil
    (i) Afferent defect
    (ii) Miosis
    (iii) Facility of dilation
    (iv) Synechiae
    (v) Iridodonesis
l. Cataract morphology and stage
m. Fundoscopy (pre and post dilatation)
n. Biometry
3. General
    a. Age
    b. Occupation
    c. Domestic circumstances
    d. Mental state
    e. Cardiovascular disorders
    f. Respiratory disorders
    g. Prostatic disorders
    h. Metabolic disorders
    i. Drug history
    j. Allergies

Indications for cataract extraction
1. Visual
2. Medical
    a. Retinal views, e.g. diabetic retinopathy
    b. Lens induced disease
3. Cosmetic

Methods of cataract extraction
1. Simple extraction
    a. Intracapsular
    b. Extracapsular
    c. Lensectomy
    d. Lens aspiration
    e. Phacoemulsification
2. Extraction with lens implantation

Causes of congenital cataracts
1. Heredity (25% of congenital cataracts). Usually autosomal dominant
2. Maternal infection, e.g. rubella, cytomegalovirus
3. Maternal drug ingestion
4. Maternal malnutrition, e.g. vitamin D deficiency
5. Metabolic disorders, e.g. galactosaemia, hypocalcaemia, amino aciduria (Lowe's syndrome)
6. Chromosomal abnormalities, e.g. Down's syndrome
7. Systemic disorders, e.g oxycephaly
8. Intraocular disease, e.g. uveitis

Management of congenital cataracts
1. Early detection and treatment important
2. Visual deprivation during sensitive period results in degeneration of lateral geniculate cells *+ Hubel - Wiesel*
3. Assessment
   a. Ocular *1ˢᵗ week or 2*
      (i) Unilateral means poorer prognosis for vision *←*
      (ii) Density of opacity *- use direct v/s indirect view.*
      (iii) Morphology related to aetiology
      (iv) Associated ocular pathology
      (v) Visual function — history, observation
                             — nystagmus (poor prognosis) ⌐
                             — specific tests, e.g. preferential looking and visual evoked potentials
   b. General
      (i) Rubella IgM titres
      (ii) Viral cultures *rubella, Cm V, TOXO*
      (iii) Urine for reducing substances and amino acid assay *Lowes*
      (iv) Blood glucose and calcium *hypogly, hypoparathyroid*
      (v) Skull X-ray *hypoparathyroid basal ganglia calcified*
4. Parents
   a. Establish any causes of cataract *- rubella, mps (steroids, Thalidom)*
   b. Motivation for care of child, e.g. contact lens wear ⌐

Bilat with bad VA - surgery immediately
* "   "   OK VA at nearest can postpone*
* "   "   develops ↓ VA etc - operate.*

Retinal detachment and vitreous disorders

Retina
1. Transparent, light-sensitive membrane
2. Lines inside of eye behind ora serrata
3. Divided into inner neurosensory layer and outer retinal pigment epithelium (RPE)

Ora serrata
1. Anterior termination of retina
2. 8 mm from nasal limbus
3. 8.5 mm from temporal limbus
4. 35 serrations interdigitate with pars plana
5. Firmly adherent to vitreous base
6. Cystic changes occur with increasing age

Bruch's membrane
1. Separates choriocapillaris from RPE
2. 5 layers
   a. Basement membrane of RPE
   b. Inner collagenous layer
   c. Elastic layer
   d. Outer collagenous layer
   e. Basement membrane of choriocapillaris

Retinal pigment epithelium
1. Features
   a. Single layer, hexagonal, epithelial cells
   b. Base in contact with Bruch's membrane
   c. Apex in contact with photoreceptors
   d. Contains melanin granules
   e. Apical zona occludens
   f. At fovea, cells taller and more numerous
   g. Cells are heaped up around optic disc
   h. In the periphery cells are larger and irregular
2. Functions
   a. Maintenance of photoreceptors
   b. Absorption of stray light

    c. Outer blood retina barrier
    d. Regeneration of visual pigment
    e. Phagocytosis
    f. Active transport of metabolites
  3. Age-related changes
    a. Thickening of basement membrane
    b. Drusen formation
    c. Macrophage invasion of drusen
    d. Loss of basal connections
    e. Cellular thinning
    f. Decreased number of nuclei
    g. Pigment clumping
  4. Embryology
    a. Develops from optic cup
    b. Pigmented between 6 and 12 weeks of gestation

Neurosensory retina
  1. Layers
    a. Outer segment of photoreceptor
    b. Outer limiting membrane and cilium of photoreceptor
    c. Outer nuclear layer (8 layers deep). Nuclei of photoreceptors
    d. Outer plexiform layers (synapse)
    e. Inner nuclear layer (5 layers deep). Nuclei of bipolar cells,
       horizontal cells, amacrine cells, Müller cells
    f. Inner plexiform layer (synapse)
    g. Ganglion cell layer
    h. Nerve fibre layer
    i. Inner limiting membrane (Müller cell end plates)
  2. Photoreceptors
     Light-sensitive cells. 2 types: rods and cones
     Rods
     120 million. 50 μm long
    a. Outer segment
        (i) Modified cilium
       (ii) Composed of 1000 stacked discs
      (iii) Discs separate from cell membrane
       (iv) Discs contain visual pigment
        (v) Discs formed at proximal end
       (vi) Shed distally in packets
      (vii) Rate of shedding 1–5/hour. Increases in light
     (viii) Total turnover in 10–14 days
    b. Cilium — microtubular structure
    c. Inner segment
        (i) Outer (ellipsoid) containing mitochondria
       (ii) Inner (myoid) containing Golgi bodies and ribosomes
    d. Outer fibre
    e. Nucleus
    f. Inner fibre

g. Synaptic region — invaginated area (triad) containing processes from bipolar and horizontal cells

Cones

6 million. 25 μm long, 85 μm long at fovea

a. Outer segment
   (i) Conical
   (ii) Stacked saccules (connected to cell membrane)
   (iii) Regenerated over 9 months
b. Cilium
c. Inner segment
d. Outer fibre
e. Nucleus
f. Inner fibre — long in foveal cones (Henle's layer)
g. Synaptic region — contains up to 20 triads

3. Modulating cells
   a. Horizontal cells
   b. Amacrine cells
4. Bipolar cells
   a. First order neurone
   b. Connect photoreceptors to ganglion cells
5. Ganglion cells
   a. 1 million (125 000 from macula)
   b. Second order neurone
   c. Connect bipolar cells to lateral geniculate body cells
   d. Large nuclei, piled 8 deep at macula
   e. Absent at fovea
   f. All or none respond to stimuli
   g. Coded response (opponent cells)
   h. At fovea — cone: ganglion cell = 1 : 1
   i. At periphery — rod: ganglion cell = 10 000 : 1
6. Müller cells
   a. Glial supporting cells
   b. Basement membrane forms inner limiting membrane
   c. Ramify widely down to outer limiting membrane
   d. Functions
      (i) Support
      (ii) Nutrition
      (iii) Ionic reservoir
      (iv) Repair (gliosis)

Embryology of retina

3 weeks — optic vesicle formed

6 weeks — optic cup formed. Initially 10 cells deep
   a. Outer layer forms RPE
   b. Inner layer forms sensory retina
   Differentiation starts at posterior pole

12 weeks — 2-layered inner retina, separated by transient fibre layer

    a. Inner neuroblastic layer develops first. Forms ganglion,
       amacrine and Müller cells
    b. Outer neuroblastic layer invades transient fibre layer. Forms
       horizontal, bipolar and photoreceptor cells
22 weeks — overall adult structure

Photochemistry
1. Visual pigments contained in photoreceptor outer segments
2. Outer segment cell membrane allows entry of sodium ions
3. Inner segment actively secretes sodium producing a current in
   the resting state (dark current)
4. Light causes changes in the pigment such that calcium ions are
   released blocking sodium channels and producing a graded
   hyperpolarization of the receptor, resulting in reduced
   neurotransmitter release

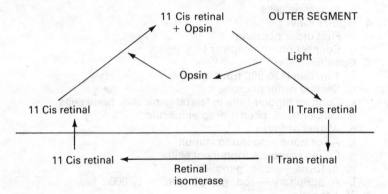

Fig. 2 The visual cycle

Response to light
1. Rod maximal at 500 nm
2. Red cone maximal at 570 nm
3. Green cone maximal at 535 nm
4. Blue cone maximal at 440 nm

Ocular sensitivity
1. Photopic maximal at 555 nm
2. Scotopic maximal at 507 nm (Purkinje shift)

Dark adaptation
Increasing ocular sensitivity with time in darkness
1. Initial faster cone adaptation
2. Slower but greater increase in rod sensitivity. Maximal at
   30–45 minutes

Retinal image
Transformation of light into membrane potentials.
Intraretinal processing
1. Primary image from photoreceptors
2. Secondary image produced in bipolars and modified by horizontal cells
3. Tertiary image produced in ganglion cells and modified by amacrine cells (opponent theory)

Colour vision
3 types of cones responding to primary colours (trichromacy theory)
Intraretinal processing occurs such that colour is coded along the yellow-blue and red-green axes

Vitreous
1. Features
   a. Virtually acellular viscous content of globe
   b. Framework of collagen fibrils reinforced with hyaluronic acid molecules
   c. 98% water
   d. Volume = 4.5 ml in emmetropic eye
   e. Cortical vitreous contains a higher concentration of collagen fibrils. Deficient over premacular and peripapillary areas
   f. Gel vitreous contains membranelles
2. Condensations
   a. Boundary
      (i) Anterior hyaloid membrane
      (ii) Posterior hyaloid membrane
   b. Central — divides gel into tracts
   c. Tubular axial tract (Cloquet's canal)
3. Attachments
   a. Vitreous base
      (i) 3–4 mm annular attachment
      (ii) Very strong
      (iii) Extends across ora serrata
   b. Weigert's ligament — 8–9 mm annular attachment to posterior lens surface (anterior end of Cloquet's canal)
   c. Vitreopapillary adhesions — at posterior end of Cloquet's canal. Visible as Weiss's ring following posterior vitreous detachment
   d. Vascular adhesions
   e. Areas of vitreoretinal degenerations, e.g. lattice degeneration, cystic retinal tufts
4. Ageing changes
   a. Dissociation of hyaluronic acid from fibrils
   b. Pooling of hyaluronic acid
   c. Fibril degeneration and reduced elasticity

   d. Drainage of hyaluronic acid into retrovitreal space
      (producing posterior vitreous detachment)
5. Function — important in oculogenesis
6. Embryology
   a. Primary vitreous
      (i) Develops at 5 weeks
      (ii) Vascularized
      (iii) Attached to optic cup and lens vesicle
   b. Secondary vitreous
      (i) Evidence at 9 weeks
      (ii) Secreted by ciliary body
      (iii) Avascular
   c. Tertiary vitreous
      (i) Develops at 24 weeks
      (ii) Forms lens zonule

Rhegmatogenous retinal detachment

Retinal detachment occuring in association with retinal hole
formation. Incidence 1 in 10 000 per year
1. Predisposing conditions
   a. Increasing age
   b. High myopia
   c. Trauma
   d. Aphakia (1% after intracapsular extraction, 0.1% after
      extracapsular extraction with intact posterior capsule)
   e. Vitreoretinal degenerations
   f. Diabetes mellitus
2. Pathogenesis of detachment
   a. Dynamic vitreoretinal traction occurs at points of abnormal
      adhesion following posterior vitreous detachment
   b. This results in transmission of energy to retina
   c. Hole formation may relieve traction
   d. Subretinal fluid may collect causing detachment
   e. Sensory retina detaches from RPE
   f. Retina becomes oedematous and opaque
   g. Photoreceptor degeneration occurs
   h. Vitreous haemorrhage may result from vascular traction
   i. RPE cells may be avulsed into vitreous causing 'tobacco
      dust' and predispose to fibrosis
3. Types of hole
   a. Horseshoe
   b. Atrophic hole
   Causes: myopia; increasing age
   c. Dialysis
      (i) Involves splitting of vitreous base
      (ii) Usually inferotemporal
      (iii) Causes: Spontaneous; Trauma

    d. Macular hole
    Causes: commotio retinae; myopia
    e. Giant retinal tear
        (i) 90 to 360° tears
        (ii) May fold back
        (iii) Associated with fibrosis,
        (iv) Causes: trauma; myopia
    f. Bucket handle tears
        (i) Avulsion of vitreous base
        (ii) Cause: trauma
4. Symptoms
    a. Photopsia
    b. Floaters
    c. Shadow
    d. 60% of patients with detachment have all these symptoms
5. Examination
    a. Visual acuity
    b. Visual fields
    c. Extent of detachment
    d. Distribution and amount of subretinal fluid
    e. Presence of 'high water' marks
    f. Position and type of retinal hole using 3-mirror contact lens
      and indentation techniques
    g. Presence of vitreoretinal traction
    h. Incidental findings
        (i) Mild anterior uveitis
        (ii) Low intraocular pressure
        (iii) Tobacco dust in vitreous
6. Natural history
    a. Total detachment
    b. Spontaneous reattachment (may occur)
    c. Retinal and RPE atrophy
    d. 'High water' mark (reactive hyperplasia of RPE at junction of
      attached retina)
    e. Viscous subretinal fluid
    f. Intraretinal cyst formation
    g. Proliferative vitreoretinopathy
    h. Rubeosis iridis
    i. Phthisis
7. Treatment principles
    a. Posturing and immobilization
    b. Re-examination
    c. Localization and closure of holes
    d. Relief of vitreoretinal traction
        (i) Scleral buckling
        (ii) Vitrectomy
    e. Production of RPE and neuroretinal adhesion
        (i) Photocoagulation
        (ii) Cryotherapy

    f. Internal tamponade
      (i) Air
      (ii) Other gases, e.g. sulphur hexafluoride
      (iii) Silicone oil
    g. Treatment of predisposing lesions in fellow eye
8. Complications of cryotherapy
    a. Proliferative vitreoretinopathy
    b. Uveitis
    c. Pigment granules in vitreous and subretinal space
    d. Cystoid macular oedema
    e. Reactive choroidal hyperaemia
    f. Intraocular haemorrhage
    g. Chorioretinal necrosis
9. Indications for drainage of subretinal fluid
    a. Large amount of subretinal fluid preventing hole localization
    b. Rigid retina
    c. Vitreous traction
    d. Longstanding detachment
    e. To allow tamponade without occluding the central retinal
      artery
10. Complications of subretinal fluid drainage
    a. Haemorrhage
    b. Retinal tear
    c. Retinal incarceration
    d. Hypotony
    e. Vitreous loss
    f. Infection
11. Complications of detachment surgery
    a. Ischaemia of anterior or posterior segments
    b. Infection
    c. Perforation
    d. Erosion of plomb into eye
    e. Extrusion of plomb
    f. Muscle imbalance
    g. Changes in refraction
    h. Macular pucker
    i. Cataract
    j. Glaucoma
    k. Redetachment

Vitreoretinal degenerations

1. Predisposing to retinal detachments
    a. Lattice degeneration — present in 40% of detached retinae
    b. Snail track degeneration
    c. White without pressure
2. Benign
    a. White with pressure
    b. Pigment clumping

   c. Diffuse chorioretinal atrophy
   d. Peripheral microcystoid changes
   e. Snowflake degeneration
   f. Pavingstone degeneration
   g. Honeycomb degeneration
   h. Drusen
   i. Oral pigmentary degeneration

Causes of traction retinal detachments
1. Penetrating ocular trauma
2. Proliferative retinopathies
   a. Diabetes mellitus
   b. Sickle cell retinopathy
   c. Retinopathy of prematurity
   d. Retinal vein occlusion
   e. Eales' disease
3. Persistent hyperplastic primary vitreous

Causes of exudative retinal detachments
1. Uveitis
2. Acute retinal necrosis
3. Choroidal tumour
   a. Malignant melanoma
   b. Metastatic
4. Glomerulonephritis (hypoproteinaemia)
5. Hypertension
6. Eclampsia
7. Hypothyroidism

Hereditary conditions associated with retinal detachments
1. Marfan's syndrome
2. Wagner's disease
3. Stickler's disease
4. Familial exudative vitreoretinopathy
5. Norrie's disease

Retinoschisis
Splits or cysts within neurosensory retinal layers
1. Senile
   Splits in outer plexiform layer
   a. Features
      (i)   Bilateral in 33%
     (ii)   Usually inferotemporal
    (iii)   Often in hypermetropia
    (iv)   Dome elevation of inner retinal layers
     (v)   White dots on inner limiting membrane
    (vi)   Beaten metal appearance of inner leaf
   (vii)   Sheathing of peripheral retinal vessels

(viii) Round holes can occur in inner leaf
(ix) Larger holes can occur in outer leaf
(x) 1% progress to rhegmatogenous retinal detachments
  b. Symptoms
     (i) Often none
     (ii) Visual field defect if posterior to equator
  c. Management
     (i) Periodic observation, e.g. field charts
     (ii) Surgery for subsequent retinal detachment
2. Juvenile
   X-linked recessive inheritance. Splits in nerve fibre layer.
   Bilateral disorder
   a. Types
      (i) Foveal
      (ii) Peripheral
   b. Associations
      (i) Goldmann-Favre disease
      (ii) Wagner's disease
   c. Management
      (i) Conservative
      (ii) Detachment surgery
      (iii) Prognosis poor
3. Secondary
   a. Causes
      (i) Proliferative retinopathies
      (ii) Trauma
      (iii) Other causes of vitreous traction
   b. Management — conservative

Vitreous opacities
1. Muscae volitantes — remnants of hyaloid system
2. Syneresis
3. Haemorrhage
4. Asteroid hyalosis
   a. Appears in 1 in 200 eyes
   b. Composed of calcium soaps adherent to fibrils
   c. Does not settle at rest
   d. Commoner in diabetics
5. Synchysis scintillans
6. Inflammatory
   a. Pars planitis
   b. Chorioretinitis
7. Neoplastic
8. Amyloid
9. Tobacco dust

Vitreous degenerations
1. Syneresis
   a. Vitreous liquefaction
   b. Aggregation and condensation of collagen fibrils
   c. Associated with floaters
   d. Causes
      (i) Myopia
      (ii) Senescence
      (iii) Trauma
      (iv) Inflammations
2. Detachment
   a. Collapse of vitreous gel
   b. Associated with floaters and photopsia
   c. May result in vitreous haemorrhage or retinal hole
      formation

Vitreous haemorrhage
1. Causes
   a. Proliferative retinopathies
      (i) Diabetes mellitus
      (ii) Retinal vein occlusion
      (iii) Sickle cell retinopathy
      (iv) Eales' disease
      (v) Retinopathy of prematurity
   b. Posterior vitreous detachment
   c. Trauma
   d. Disciform macular degeneration
   e. Blood dyscrasias
   f. Subarachnoid haemorrhage (Terson's syndrome)
2. Complications
   a. Syneresis
   b. Inflammation and fibrosis — leads to traction detachment
   c. Haemosiderosis
   d. Glaucoma, haemolytic or ghost cell
   e. Synchysis scintillans — cholesterol crystals. Settle inferiorly
      at rest
   f. Ochre membrane

Persistent hyperplastic primary vitreous
1. Anterior (90%)
   a. Unilateral retrolental mass
   b. Elongated ciliary processes
   c. Microphthalmos
   d. Cataract ←
   e. Secondary angle closure glaucoma   due to lens swe...
   f. Vitreous haemorrhage

2. Posterior (10%)
   a. White membrane from optic disc to peripheral retina. Usually inferior
   b. Tractional retinal detachment
   c. 'Morning Glory' syndrome may be a variant

Causes of leukocoria (white pupil, cat's eye pupil)
1. Cataract
2. Retrolental masses
   a. Persistent hyperplastic primary vitreous
   b. Retinopathy of prematurity
   c. Norrie's disease
3. Tumours
   a. Retinoblastoma
   b. Choroidal metastases
4. Exudates
   a. Familial exudative vitreoretinopathy
   b. Coats' disease
   c. Eales' disease
5. Change in retina or choroid
   a. Incontinentia pigmentii
   b. High myopia
   c. Myelinated nerve fibres (extensive)
   d. Retinal dysplasia
   e. Choroideraemia
6. Infections
   a. Toxoplasmosis
   b. Toxocariasis
   c. Endophthalmitis

Indications for vitrectomy
1. Anterior segment conditions
   a. Accidental vitreous loss during surgery
   b. Lensectomy, e.g. for secondary cataract in childhood arthritis
   c. Excision of pupillary membranes
   d. Vitreous touch causing bullous keratopathy
   e. Incarceration of vitreous in cataract section
   f. Malignant (ciliary block) glaucoma
   g. Blockage of trabeculectomy or drainage tube
2. Posterior segment conditions
   a. Persistent vitreous opacity
      (i) Haemorrhage
      (ii) Vitreous membranes
      (iii) Amyloidosis
   b. Advanced diabetic eye disease
   c. Penetrating trauma
   d. Retained intraocular foreign bodies

e. Preretinal membranes
f. Proliferative vitreoretinopathy
g. Complicated retinal detachments, e.g. giant tears
h. Endophthalmitis
i. Persistent hyperplastic primary vitreous
j. Vitreous biopsy

Retinal vascular disorders

BLOOD SUPPLY TO RETINA

1. Central retinal artery
   a. First branch of ophthalmic artery
   b. True artery
   c. End artery
   d. Divides into upper and lower trunks usually at optic disc
   e. Accompanied by vein
2. Retinal arteries
   a. Subdivisions of trunks
   b. 2 superior and 2 inferior
   c. Histologically arterioles with little elastic tissue
   d. Surrounded by capillary free zone (120 μm)
3. Cilioretinal artery
   a. Present in 20% of patients
   b. Supply from posterior ciliary circulation
   c. Supplies variable area of retina
4. Capillaries
   a. Lined by non-fenestrated endothelium
   b. Capillary walls contain pericytes
   c. 2 plexi
      (i) Deep
      (ii) Superficial
   d. Absent from foveal avascular zones
5. Retinal veins
   a. Main branches mirror arterioles
   b. Drain to central retinal vein
   c. Share common sheath at arteriovenous crossings
   d. Normal artery : vein diameter ratio = 2 : 3
6. Vascular anomalies
   a. Divisions into main arterioles may occur on disc or a little way into the retina
   b. Anomalous trifurcations associated with disc drusen
   c. Congenital tortuosity

PHYSIOLOGY

1. Central retinal artery
   a. Arterial pressure $\simeq$ 75 mmHg
   b. Arterial pulsations occur if blood pressure < intraocular pressure
2. Capillaries
   a. Pressure $\simeq$ 55 mmHg
   b. Retinal artery–capillary pressure drop due to increased surface area
   c. Absent precapillary sphincters
   d. All capillary beds perfused
   e. Capillary endothelial tight junctions account for blood retinal barrier
   f. Capillaries impermeable to proteins ensuring little extracellular fluid of low osmotic pressure
3. Central retinal vein
   Pressure $\simeq$ 25 mmHg
4. Retinal perfusion
   Relates to
   a. Vascular pressure head
   b. Vascular resistance
   c. Blood viscosity
5. Autoregulation of retinal flow
   a. Ensures adequate perfusion over range of intraocular pressures
   b. No neurogenic control
   c. Some chemical control
      (High Po_2 producing constriction; High Pco_2 producing dilatation)

EMBRYOLOGY

1. Retina initially avascular
2. Retinal arterioles develop as branches of hyaloid artery
3. Extend to equator by 8 months
4. Temporal retina may not be vascularized at birth
5. Capillaries penetrate to inner nuclear layer
6. Central retinal vein develops by 3 months
7. Vascular pattern not genetically determined

DIABETES MELLITUS

1. Disorder of glucose metabolism due to diminished availability or effectiveness of insulin
2. Results in an increase in blood glucose concentration
3. Random blood glucose of > 11.0 mmol/l or fasting blood glucose of > 8 mmol/l

4. In Great Britain 1–2% of the population. 500 000 cases diagnosed and possibly 500 000 undiagnosed

Types
1. Juvenile onset insulin dependent diabetes (Type I)
   a. Often presents acutely with systemic disease: fatigue, weight loss, polyuria, polydipsia, infection and coma
   b. Multifactorial aetiology
      (i) Viruses (especially Coxsackie B4)
      (ii) Genetic predisposition (associated with HLA-DR3, DR4, B8 and B15)
      (iii) Pancreatic islet cell antibodies
   c. Peak incidence between 11 and 14 years of age
2. Mature onset non-insulin dependent (Type II)
   a. Tends to occur in the elderly and overweight
   b. Often asymptomatic
   c. Probably inherited. Nearly all identical twins with Type II diabetes mellitus have a similarly affected co-twin
   d. Occurs most frequently between the ages of 50 and 70 years
3. Secondary
   a. Drugs
      (i) Steroids
      (ii) Thiazide diuretics
   b. Endocrine
      (i) Acromegaly
      (ii) Cushing's
      (iii) Thyrotoxicosis
   c. Pancreatic, e.g. pancreatitis

Features
1. Vascular
   a. Large vessel disease, e.g. myocardial infarction
   b. Small vessel disease, e.g. renal failure, gangrene.
2. Renal
   a. Diffuse glomerulosclerosis and nodular glomerulosclerosis (Kimmelstiel-Wilson lesion)
   b. Pyelonephritis and renal papillary necrosis
3. Neuromuscular
   Mononeuritis, peripheral neuropathy, autonomic neuropathy and amyotrophy (painful, asymetrical weakness and wasting of quadriceps)
4. Skin
   a. Sensitivity and lipoatrophy at injection sites.
   b. Necrobiosis lipoidica diabeticorum over shins
5. Infections, e.g. candida and tuberculosis
6. Ocular
   a. Blepharitis, styes
   b. Recurrent corneal erosions

    c. Iris
      (i) Neuropathy (poor dilatation)
      (ii) Pigment loss
      (iii) Neovascularization and secondary glaucoma
    d. Chronic open angle glaucoma
    e. Cataracts
    f. Refractive changes in lens (hypermetropia > myopia)
    g. Retinopathy
    h. Vitreous haemorrhage
    i. Ischaemic optic neuropathy
    j. Cranial nerve palsies, e.g. 3rd nerve

DIABETIC RETINOPATHY

1. Prevalence of retinopathy at time of diagnosis — 1.5% age 20–40 years; 7% age 50–60 years; 10% in older patients
2. Retinopathy at diagnosis is probably the result of a long period of undiagnosed and often asymptomatic hyperglycaemia in middle aged and elderly diabetics
3. Prevalence of retinopathy rises with duration of disease to a peak of 80–85% after 20 years after diagnosis
4. Diabetic retinopathy is the commonest cause of blind and partial sight registration in the 30–60 year age group (U.K.)
5. 50% of blind diabetics are dead within 3–4 years of registration and only 20% survive for 10 years

Possible factors in the pathogenesis of diabetic retinopathy
1. Thickening of basement membrane with deposits of glycogen and carbohydrate
2. Capillary endothelial cell damage
3. Biochemical changes in red blood cells leading to defective oxygen transport
4. Increased stickiness and aggregation of platelets
5. Loss of vascular pericytes

Classification
1. Background
2. Maculopathy
    a. Exudative
    b. Oedematous
    c. Ischaemic
    d. Mixed
3. Pre-proliferative
4. Proliferative
5. Advanced diabetic eye disease
    a. Persistent vitreous haemorrhage
    b. Retinal detachment
    c. Opaque membrane formation
    d. Neovascular glaucoma

Signs of background diabetic retinopathy
1. Microaneurysms
   a. First clinically detectable changes of diabetic retinopathy
   b. Inner nuclear layer of the retina
2. Hard exudates
   Outer plexiform and inner nuclear layers
3. Haemorrhages
   a. Flame-shaped — retinal nerve fibre layer
   b. Dot and blot — middle retinal layers

Diabetic maculopathy
1. Retinopathy in the macula area
2. Commonest cause of visual loss in patients with diabetes mellitus
3. More common in type II diabetics

Classification
1. Exudative
   a. Features
      (i) Exudates in the macula area
      (ii) Circinate rings
   b. Management
      (i) Photocoagulation may be beneficial when vision is better than 6/60
      (ii) Treatment to centre of circinate rings
2. Oedematous
   a. Features
      (i) Macular oedema
      (ii) Extracellular fluid in Henle's layer. May be seen by microscopic examination of the macular area or on fluorescein angiography
   b. Management
      (i) Macular grid with low intensity, short duration laser
      (ii) Laser before vision worse than 6/18
3. Ischaemic
   a. Features
      Fluorescein angiogram reveals capillary non-perfusion
   b. Management
      (i) No proven treatment
      (ii) 30% proceed to proliferative diabetic retinopathy within 2 years so may eventually require panretinal photocoagulation
4. Mixed
   a. Features
      (i) Exudates
      (ii) Ischaemia
      (iii) Oedema
   b. Management
      Photocoagulation may be of benefit

Preproliferative diabetic retinopathy
1. Features
   a. Cotton wool spots
   b. Venous changes — dilatation and beading of the vessels
   c. Arteriolar narrowing
   d. Large blotch haemorrhages
   e. Intraretinal microvascular abnormalities (IRMA)
   f. Capillary closure on fluorescein angiogram
2. Management
   Photocoagulation as high risk of proliferative diabetic
   retinopathy

Proliferative diabetic retinopathy
1. Incidence
   a. Overall incidence of proliferative change 10–20%
   b. Incidence greater for insulin dependent diabetics than for
      non-insulin dependent diabetics
2. Pathogenesis
   a. Extensive retinal capillary closure
   b. Angiogenesis factor release stimulates proliferation
   c. Endothelial buds from the venous end of capillaries
   d. Fibrovascular network adherent to vitreous face
   e. Vitreous detachment may elevate vessels
   f. New vessels bleed resulting in further vitreous contraction
      and retinal detachment
3. Features
   a. Neovascularization — this is essential for the diagnosis of
      proliferative diabetic retinopathy. It occurs at the disc (NVD)
      or elsewhere (NVE)
   b. Fibrovascular epiretinal membrane — Initially transparent
      but becomes opaque
   c. Vitreous traction with retinal detachment
4. Prognosis

Table 4

	If untreated risk of severe visual loss in 2 years	If treated with photocoagulation risk of severe visual loss in 2 years
a. Severe NVD, vitreous haemorrhage	40%	20%
b. Moderate to severe NVD, no vitreous haemorrhage	25%	5%
c. NVE, vitreous haemorrhage	30%	7%
d. NVE, no vitreous haemorrhage	7%	7%

5. Management
   a. Photocoagulation
   b. Ensure good control of blood glucose levels. Retinopathy
      may worsen temporarily if control suddenly improves
   c. Stop smoking
   d. Treat systemic hypertension
   e. Avoid heavy physical exertion or strain
   f. Avoid rapid changes in blood glucose levels
   g. Avoid direct trauma
   h. Reduce heavy alcohol consumption

Photocoagulation in proliferative diabetic retinopathy
1. Indications
   a. New vessels at the disc (NVD), especially if there has been
      vitreous haemorrhage
   b. New vessels elsewhere (NVE) with vitreous haemorrhage
   c. New vessels elsewhere or ischaemic changes (if the patient
      cannot be followed up reliably)
2. Technique
   a. Contact lenses — fundus contact lens for macular view, 3
      mirror contact lens for peripheral photocoagulation.
      Panfunduscopic lens gives a wider field of vision but
      inverted image like indirect ophthalmoscope
   b. Mild flat NVE — blanch retinal pigment epithelium.
      200–500 μm spot size. 0.02–0.20 seconds (Argon laser)
   c. Elevated NVE — may be necessary to treat vessels directly.
      Often reopen after treatment. May bleed
   d. Moderate to severe NVE — panretinal photocoagulation
      with 2000–3500 burns. 500 μ spot size. 0.02–0.20 seconds
   e. NVD — panretinal photocoagulation

Advanced diabetic eye disease
1. Clinical features
   a. Persistent vitreous haemorrhage
   b. Tractional retinal detachment
      Types:
      (i) Tangential
      (ii) Anteroposterior
      (iii) Bridging traction
   c. Opaque membrane on posterior hyaloid face
   d. Neovascular glaucoma with rubeosis iridis
2. Management
   a. Vitrectomy
   b. Cutting of traction membranes
   c. Epiretinal membrane peeling
   d. Endolaser
   e. Atropine, steroids and eventually retrobulbar alcohol and
      enucleation for a painful blind eye

HYPERTENSION

1. Definitions (WHO)
   a. Normotension — systolic ≤140
                     — diastolic ≤90
   b. Borderline   — systolic >140–<160 mmHg
                     — diastolic >90–<95
   c. Hypertension — systolic ≥160
                     — diastolic ≥95
2. Causes
   a. Essential (95%)
   b. Renal disease
   c. Endocrine disease, e.g. Cushing's syndrome, Conn's syndrome, phaeochromocytoma, acromegaly
   d. Contraceptive pill and eclampsia
   e. Coarctation of the aorta
3. Histopathology
   a. 'Benign' hypertension
      (i) Arteriole hyalinization. Deposits of eosinophilic material under endothelium and eventually in vessel wall
      (ii) Small/medium sized arteries. Medial muscular hypertrophy and fibrosis with intimal proliferation. Micro-aneurysm formation in small perforating arteries of the brain
      (iii) Large arteries. Accelerated atherosclerosis
   b. 'Malignant' hypertension
      Arterioles. Endothelial damage allowing red blood cells and plasma to leak into vessel wall where fibrin precipitates = 'fibrinoid necrosis' of the arteriolar wall. Focal spasm and segmental dilatation.
4. Complications
   a. Left ventricular failure
   b. Renal failure
   c. Strokes and hypertensive encephalopathy
   d. Myocardial infarction
   e. Complications of treatment
   f. Retinopathy
5. Ocular features
   a. Vaso-constriction with arteriolar narrowing
   b. Leakage leading to haemorrhages, retinal oedema and exudates
   c. Exudates may deposit radially around the fovea in Henle's layer (macular star)
   d. Cotton wool spots
6. Grading of hypertensive retinopathy
   Grade 1 — silver wiring
   Grade 2 — arteriovenous nipping
   Grade 3 — grade 2 and haemorrhages, exudates and cotton wool spots
   Grade 4 — changes of grade 3 and disc swelling. The general prognosis is the same with grade 3 or grade 4 changes

Signs of arteriosclerotic retinopathy
Usually associated with hypertension
1. Arteriovenous nipping (Salus' sign)
2. Dilated vein distal to arterio-venous crossing (Bonnet's sign)
3. Tapering of vein on either side of crossing (Gunn's sign)
4. Right angle deflection of vein
5. Silver wiring of arterioles
6. Ischaemic choroidal infarcts (Elschnig's spots)
7. Retinal arterial macroaneurysm
8. Ischaemic optic neuropathy

Macular star
Star-shaped exudates in Henle's layer of the macula
Causes
1. Hypertension
2. Papilloedema
3. Papillitis —
4. Ocular or cerebral trauma
5. Obstruction of arteries or veins supplying macular area
6. Retinal periphlebitis
7. Juxtapapillary choroiditis
8. Chronic infections, e.g. tuberculosis, syphilis
9. Idiopathic

— Neuroretinits (Lebers stellate maculop — NO MS asso

Cotton wool spots
1. White, fluffy, retinal lesions
2. Represent areas of retinal ischaemia which cause disruption of axonal transport
3. Axonal swelling and rupture
4. Products of axonal transport accumulate at end of axon resulting in 'cytoid bodies'

Causes
1. Malignant hypertension
2. Diabetic retinopathy
3. Anaemia
4. Infective conditions, e.g. septicaemia, subacute bacterial endocarditis, acquired immune defiency syndrome
5. Collagen vascular diseases, e.g. Lupus erythematosus, polyarteritis nodosa
6. Retinopathy following crush injuries (Purtscher's retinopathy)

Retinal macroaneurysm
1. Features
   a. Occurs in elderly, hypertensive or arteriosclerotic individuals
   b. Single or multiple
   c. Usually at posterior pole

d. May subsequently
   (i) Occlude spontaneously
   (ii) Bleed
   (iii) Leak — circinate exudate
        — macular oedema
2. Management
   a. Conservative
   b. Photocoagulation

RETINAL VEIN OCCLUSION

BRVO → hemi, macula, etc.
CRVO → Non-isch → venous stasis
→ isch → many cws, ⊕ blood!!
→ papillophlebitis - young - good VA! no Tx

1. Causes *√ IVFA·*
   a. Pressure on the vein
      (i) Systemic hypertension with arterial pressure on vein
          (artery and vein share common fibrous sheath)
      (ii) Raised intraocular pressure *- POAG*
   b. Vessel wall disease
      (i) Diabetes
      (ii) Vessel wall inflammation, e.g. sarcoid and Behçet's *Lues.*
           disease *, sichle cell disease·*
   c. Increased blood viscosity *- due to ↑cells, ↑Proteins·*
      (i) Polycythaemia
      (ii) Leukaemia *chronic - large #s of cells!!*
      (iii) Myeloma
      (iv) Hyperlipidaemia *, Waldenstrom macrogl·, contraceptives*
2. Clinical features *— ↑Opt-ociliary sh. vessels!!*
   a. Dilated veins
   b. Flame-shaped haemorrhages
   c. Retinal oedema
   d. Cotton wool spots
   e. Venous and occasionally arterial sheathing *Late!*
   f. Exudates *- Late'. - Late → collaterals/shunts, RPE D',*
3. Complications
   a. Macular oedema *— c'*
   b. New vessel formation on the optic disc, retina and also the
      iris causing secondary glaucoma ('hundred day' glaucoma)
   c. Neovascularization may lead to vitreous haemorrhage and
      tractional retinal detachment
4. Management *S.P.*
   a. Exclude underlying cause *- √CBC, BS, electroph?, ANA, ESR, PTA/.*
   b. Photocoagulation if marked ischaemia or neovascularization *CRVO→*
      √pt g 3 weeks are present *, ...*
   c. Drugs which inhibit coagulation (unproven)
   BRVO study → Tx ① chronic mac. oed. >6 mths., ② NV → Argon G,
   CRVO. VA < 20/40· Avoid FA- Grid to Arcade
   Not

Causes of dilated retinal veins
1. Congenital, e.g. von Hippel-Lindau disease
2. Trauma and inflammation, e.g. carotico-cavernous fistula,

periphlebitis, anterior uveitis, impending obstruction of the central retinal vein
3. Cardiovascular disease
4. Respiratory disease
5. Central nervous system disease, e.g. papilloedema, subarachnoid haemorrhage
6. Haematological diseases, e.g. polycythaemia, leukaemia, myeloma
7. Febrile illnesses, e.g. septicaemia
8. Metabolic diseases, e.g. diabetic retinopathy
9. Collagen vascular diseases, e.g. polyarteritis nodosa
10. Toxic conditions, e.g. methyl alcohol ingestion

Causes of retinal vascular tortuosity
1. Normal variation
2. Congenital
3. Haematological disorders, e.g. polycythaemia, myeloma, cryoglobulinaemia and sickle cell disease
4. Hypertension
5. Haemangioma of retina
6. Hereditary haemorrhagic telangiectasia
7. Eales' disease
8. Fabry's disease
9. Coat's disease
10. Chronic open angle glaucoma

Causes of juxtafoveolar retinal telangiectasis
1. Small branch vein occlusion
2. Diabetes mellitus
3. Radiotherapy
4. Carotid artery obstruction
5. Hereditary haemorrhagic telangiectasia (Osler-Weber-Rendu syndrome)
6. Fevers
7. Cardiovascular shock
8. Anti-coagulant drug therapy
9. Intracranial haemorrhage
10. Haematological disorders
11. Trauma
12. Valsalva haemorrhagic retinopathy
13. Idiopathic

RETINAL ARTERY OCCLUSION
1. Causes
   a. External pressure, e.g raised intraocular pressure from acute closed angle glaucoma or retinal detachment surgery

   b. Vessel wall occlusion
      (i) atheroma
      (ii) arteritis, e.g. giant cell arteritis, polyarteritis nodosa, systemic lupus erythematosus
   c. Embolisation
      (i) Carotid (usually originates from bifurcation)
      (ii) Valve disease, e.g. subacute bacterial endocarditis or stenotic lesions
      (iii) Cardiac wall problems, e.g. mural thrombus from myocardial infarction, atrial myxoma
2. Types of embolus
   a. Cholesterol (Hollenhorst plaques). Atheromatous plaques appear as refractile crystals
   b. Fibrinoplatelet — cause amaurosis fugax
   c. Calcific — may cause permanent occlusion of vessel
3. Clinical features
   a. Sudden loss of vision
   b. Painless
   c. Field defect if branch occlusion
   d. Afferent pupillary defect
   e. White and oedematous retina with reflex from choroidal vessels showing through at the macula (cherry-red spot). Disappears after a few weeks
   f. 4% develop new vessels on the iris (rubeosis iridis)
   g. Optic atrophy with no other features
4. Management
   a. Acute
      (i) Ocular massage
      (ii) Intravenous acetazolamide
      (iii) Anterior chamber paracentesis
      (iv) Inhalation of high oxygen/high carbon dioxide mixture
      (v) Supine positioning of patient
   b. Exclude underlying causes particularly giant cell arteritis

Causes of a cherry-red spot
1. Central retinal artery occlusion
2. Sphingolipidoses, e.g. Tay-Sachs, Niemann-Pick, Gaucher's disease
3. Quinine toxicity
4. Traumatic retinal oedema
5. Macula retinal hole with surrounding detachment

SICKLE CELL DISEASE

Sickle cell disease is due to the presence of one or more abnormal haemoglobins causing blood cells to adopt an abnormal shape under conditions of low oxygen tension and acidosis. These deformed red blood cells cause a change in blood flow and hypoxia

1. Types
   a. AS (sickle cell trait) — requires hypoxia or abnormal conditions to produce sickling. Mild form
   b. SS (sickle cell disease) — severe systemic complications, mild ocular disease
   c. SC (sickle cell haemoglobin C disease) — severe ocular disease
   d. S Thal (sickle cell haemoglobin with thalassaemia) — severe systemic and ocular disease
2. General features
   a. Painful crises — due to tissue infarction. Precipitated by infection, dehydration and low temperature
   b. Aplastic crises — falling haemoglobin level caused by parvovirus B19 infection
   c. Sequestration crises — pooling of sickled erythrocytes in spleen, liver or lungs
   d. Infection — particularly pneumococcal. Also salmonella osteomyelitis
   e. Renal damage
   f. Chronic leg ulceration
   g. Aseptic bone necrosis
3. Ocular features
   a. Conjunctiva — dark red vascular segments shaped like commas or corkscrews. Involve small calibre vessels
   b. Iris
      (i) Focal ischaemic atrophy
      (ii) Rubeosis (rare)
      (iii) Hyphaema
   c. Retina/choroid
      (i) Venous tortuosity
      (ii) Black sun-bursts (peripheral, choroidoretinal scars)
      (iii) Salmon-patch haemorrhages (peripheral, pink, superficial haemorrhages)
      (iv) Refractile spots ← Hemosiderin deposits
      (v) Silver wiring of peripheral arterioles
      (vi) Retinal breaks
      (vii) Angioid streaks -
      (viii) Vascular occlusions — central retinal artery
                                  — macular artery
                                  — retinal vein
                                  — choroid
      (ix) Retinopathy
4. Stages of proliferative sickle retinopathy
   Stage 1 — peripheral arterial occlusions
   Stage 2 — peripheral arterio-anastomoses (dilated pre-existent capillary channel)

Stage 3 — new vessels from anastomoses ('sea-fan' neovascularization)
Stage 4 — vitreous haemorrhage
Stage 5 — vitreous traction and retinal detachment
5. Management of sickle cell retinopathy
   a. Photocoagulation
   b. Vitrectomy (late stage of proliferative disease)
   c. Retinal detachment surgery — may be complicated by anterior segment ischaemia and require exchange transfusion

Causes of retinal fan-shaped neovascularization (sea-fan)
1. Haemoglobinopathy
2. Retinopathy of prematurity (retro-lental fibroplasia)
3. Diabetes mellitus
4. Eales' disease
5. Sarcoidosis
6. Central and branch retinal vein occlusion
7. Uveitis
8. Familial exudative vitreoretinopathy

RETINOPATHY OF PREMATURITY (RETROLENTAL FIBROPLASIA)
1. Definition — a proliferative retinopathy affecting premature infants. Sometimes associated with exposure to high ambient oxygen concentrations
2. Features
   a. Active disease
      Stage 1a — spasm of retinal vessels
      Stage 1b — arterio-venous shunt (silver grey line)
      Stage 2 — dilated and tortuous veins. Intravitreal vascularization. Intraretinal haemorrhages
      Stage 3 — vitreous haemorrhage. Vitreous traction. Localized tractional retinal detachment. May still spontaneously resolve
      Stage 4 — vitreous haemorrhage. Extensive retinal detachment. Advanced proliferation
      Stage 5 — total detachment with retrolental mass. White pupil
   b. Cicatrical disease
      Grade 1 — vitroretinal membranes. High myopia common
      Grade 2 — retinal traction. May be macular displacement
      Grade 3 — falciform retinal fold
      Grade 4 — incomplete retrolental mass. Traction retinal detachment
      Grade 5 — complete retrolental mass. Organized retinal detachment. Secondary angle closure glaucoma

3. Management
   a. Monitor arterial oxygen (but may develop without exposure
      to high O$_2$ levels)
   b. Cryotherapy ⟵⟶ *5 hrs or 8 total of stg 3+*
   c. Vitamin E *?*
   d. Photocoagulation
   e. Scleral buckling — *repair any RD!!* (stg 4)

f/u q 2 whs. Per 1-2 mths
(q 1 week if any ROP found)

EALES' DISEASE
White man. Sickle cell.

Retinal periphlebitis of unknown aetiology. Affects young men.
Bilateral
1. Clinical features
   a. Recurrent vitreous haemorrhages
   b. Rubeosis iridis
   c. Neovascular glaucoma
   d. Cataract
2. Stages
   Stage 1 — sheathing of retinal venules by inflammatory
   deposits, retinal oedema and small retinal haemorrhages
   Stage 2 — more severe involvement extending into posterior
   pole with vitreous haze
   Stage 3 — peripheral retinal neovascularization
   Stage 4 — proliferative retinopathy with retinal and vitreous
   haemorrhage and tractional retinal detachment
3. Management
   a. Destroy new vessels and areas of retinal ischaemia
   b. Vitrectomy in certain cases

COATS' DISEASE   *— Leukocoria —*   *— Juxtafoveal Telang.*
                                          — Lebers miliary aneurysm
1. Clinical features
   a. Unilateral -
   b. Males in first decade
   c. Peripheral telangiectatic and aneurysmal lesions ✓✓
   d. Massive subretinal exudation resulting in
      (i) Cataract
      (ii) Glaucoma
      (iii) Retinal detachment
2. Management
   a. Photocoagulation *) be aggressive to prevent RD ✓✓.*
   b. Cryotherapy
   c. Retinal detachment surgery

Macula

Macula

1. Horizontally oval, 5 mm in diameter
2. Centre 4 mm temporal, 0.8 mm inferior to disc
3. Contains more than one ganglion cell layer
4. Xanthophyll pigment in inner retinal layers
5. Specialized areas
   a. Fovea
      (i) 1.5 mm diameter (5' of arc)
      (ii) 6–8 ganglion cell layers
      (iii) Thickened internal limiting membrane
      (iv) Retinal pigment epithelial cells taller, more numerous and contain more melanosomes
   b. Foveola
      (i) 0.26 mm diameter (54" of arc)
      (ii) Thinnest part of retina
      (iii) Central umbo responsible for foveolar reflection
      (iv) Contains only cones (150 000/mm^2)
      (v) Cones taller and thinner than elsewhere
      (vi) Inner retinal elements displaced laterally
      (vii) Cone inner fibres run parallel to retinal surface in Henle's layer with relatively little supporting structure
      (viii) Thinned internal limiting membrane
   c. Foveal avascular zone
      (i) 0.5 mm diameter
      (ii) Surrounded by continuous capillary network
      (iii) Extent visible only on fluorescein angiography

Symptoms of macular disease

1. Poor vision (especially reading)
2. Central scotoma
3. Hypermetropia (+1.0 D lens test)
4. Metamorphopsia
5. Micropsia and macropsia
6. Colour vision defects (red–green)

Examination of a patient with macular disease
1. Vision (near and distance)
2. Colour vision, e.g. colour desaturation
3. Photostress test
4. Amsler grid
5. Maddox rod
6. Perimetry
7. Fundal examination (Hruby, contact lens, +90 dioptre lens)
8. Fluorescein angiography
9. Entoptic phenomena, e.g. flying corpuscle
10. Contrast sensitivity
11. Flicker fusion frequency
12. Electrophysiological tests

Fluorescein angiography
1. Principles
   a. Excitation of fluorescein at 490 nm (blue)
   b. Fluorescent emission at 530 nm (green)
   c. Fluorescein remains intravascular within the retina but leaks from the choroidal circulation
   d. 70–80% of fluorescein protein bound
   e. 20–30% free fluorescein
2. Technique
   a. 5 mls of 10% fluorescein injected intravenously
   b. 3 mls of 25% fluorescein if media hazy
   c. Arm to eye time approximately 9 seconds
3. Phases
   a. Pre-arterial — choroidal flush
   b. Arterial — 1 second later
   c. Capillary — complete arterial and capillary filling with venous lamina flow
   d. Venous
      (i) Early
      (ii) Mid
      (iii) Late
4. Side effects (Incidence of side effects constant with differing concentrations)
   a. Yellow discolouration of skin
   b. Dark urine
   c. Nausea and vomiting
   d. Red after-image
   e. Phlebitis
   f. Syncope
   g. Laryngeal oedema
   h. Anaphylactic shock

Other uses of fluorescein
1. Detection of corneal epithelial defects

2. Applanation tonometry
3. Tear film assessment
4. Hard contact lens fitting
5. Test of lacrimal drainage system patency
6. Seidel's test for aqueous leakage
7. Anterior segment angiography
8. Fluorophotometry

Causes of hyperfluorescence
1. Atrophy of RPE cells (window defect)
2. Dye in subretinal space
3. Dye in RPE detachment
4. Dye leakage from retinal vessels
5. Dye leakage from choroidal or retinal new vessels
6. Dye leakage from optic nerve head in papilloedema
7. Staining of tissues by dye, e.g. drusen

Causes of hypofluorescence
1. Masking by abnormal materials, e.g. blood, melanin and hard
   exudates
2. Ischaemia of retinal vessels
3. Ischaemia of choroidal vessels
4. Atrophy of vascular tissue, e.g. myopia

Senile macular degeneration (SMD)
Leading cause of blindness in the western world. Accounts for
26–30% of all blind registrations in the United Kingdom. Bilateral
asymmetrical disease
1. Drusen
   a. White–yellow lesions at posterior pole
   b. Occur frequently in patients over 60 years
   c. Composed of hyaline material deposited in Bruch's
      membrane
   d. May represent reduced efficiency of RPE phagocytosis
   e. 2 morphological types
      (i) Large, fluffy
      (ii) Small, discrete
   f. Associated with
      (i) Atrophy of RPE and photoreceptor outer segments
      (ii) Thickening of Bruch's membrane
      (iii) Macrophage invasion of drusen
      (iv) Neovascular membrane proliferation
2. Dry SMD
   a. Choroidal sclerosis
   b. Large areas of well-circumscribed atrophy of RPE,
      neurosensory retina and choriocapillaris
   c. Large choroidal vessels prominent

3. Exudative (wet) SMD
   Two forms
   a. Retinal pigment epithelial detachment
      (i) Dome-shaped elevation
      (ii) Fluid derived from choriocapillaris
      (iii) May resolve
      (iv) 66% develop SRNVM
   b. Subretinal neovascular membrane (SRNVM)
      (i) Exudative detachment of RPE or retina
      (ii) Haemorrhage — sub RPE, sub retinal, vitreous
      (iii) Disciform scarring

Disciform degeneration
Circumscribed scarring at macula as a result of haemorrhage from
subretinal neovascular membranes. Subretinal neovascular
membranes are stimulated to proliferate as a result of
abnormalities of choriocapillaris, Bruch's membrane, RPE and
outer retinal layers.

Causes of subretinal neovascular membranes (SRNVM)
1. Congenital or hereditary
   a. Rubella retinopathy
   b. Best's disease
   c. Cone dystrophy
   d. Retinitis pigmentosa
2. Inflammatory
   a. Acute multifocal placoid pigment epitheliopathy
   b. Harada's disease
   c. Presumed ocular histoplasmosis syndrome
   d. Chronic uveitis
   e. Toxoplasmosis
   f. Toxocara
3. Vascular
   a. Coats' disease
   b. Central or branch retinal vein occlusion
4. Traumatic
   a. Choroidal rupture
   b. Photocoagulation
   c. Retinal detachment surgery
5. Neoplastic
   a. Choroidal naevus
   b. Choroidal melanoma
   c. Choroidal haemangioma
   d. Choroidal metastases
   e. RPE hamartoma
6. Degenerative
   a. Senile macular degeneration
   b. Myopia (Fuch's spot)

        c. Angioid streaks
        d. Serpiginous choroidopathy
        e. Optic nerve drusen

Management of SMD
    1. Observe, especially if fellow eye blind
    2. Low vision aids
    3. Blind/partial sight registration
    4. Photocoagulation if SRNVM is present. Reasonable chance of
       benefit if
        a. Vision 6/18 or better
        b. Duration of symptoms less than one month
        c. Neovascular membrane more than 200 μm from foveola

Angioid streaks
Dehiscences in collagenous and elastic layers of Bruch's
membrane, with secondary changes in choriocapillaris and RPE
    1. Features
        a. Dark irregular lines radiating from optic disc
        b. May interlink around the optic disc
        c. Irregular paths ending abruptly posterior to the equator
        d. May cause subretinal neovascularization
        e. Usually bilateral
        f. 50% related to systemic disorders of skin, bone and blood
    2. Associations
        a Pseudoxanthoma elasticum
        b. Ehlers-Danlos syndrome
        c. Marfan's syndrome
        d. Paget's disease
        e. Sickle cell disease
        f. Thalassaemia
        g. Lead poisoning
        h. Acromegaly

"PEPSI" P E P S I V   *I Idiopthic 50%.*

Central serous choroidoretinopathy
    1. Features
        a. Unilateral
        b. Males > females, 20–45 years
        c. Often 'dynamic' personality types
        d. Myopic
    2. Symptoms
        a. Blurring of central vision
        b. Metamorphopsia
        c. Micropsia
    3. Signs
        a. Visual acuity 6/6 to 6/36. Often improves with a +1.00 D
           lens
        b. Positive paracentral or central scotoma

    c. Red desaturation
    d. Small serous sensory retinal detachment of macula
    e Sometimes in association with optic disc pit
4. Pathogenesis
    a. Breakdown of outer blood-retinal barrier
    b. Fluid in subretinal space
    c. Sometimes associated with a smaller RPE detachment
5. Fluorescein angiogram — smokestack or inkblot appearance in late venous phase
6. Prognosis
    a. 90% spontaneously resolve
    b. 40% recur
7. Treatment
    a. Conservative
    b. Photocoagulation if
       (i) recurrences have left a visual defect
      (ii) duration is longer than 6 months
     (iii) visual impairment in affected fellow eye

Cystoid macular oedema
1. Features
    a. Lack of supporting mechanisms for Henle's layer allows accumulation of extracellular fluid leaking from macular capillaries
    b. Forms flower-petal arrangement due to radiation of cone fibres
    c. May develop intraretinal cysts *of outer plexiform layer?*
2. Causes
    a. Vitreous
       (i) Preretinal membrane formation
      (ii) Vitritis
    b. Retina
       (i) Diabetes
      (ii) Central or branch retinal vein occlusion
     (iii) Macroaneurysms
     (iv) Telangiectasia
      (v) Hypertension
     (vi) Tumours
    (vii) Retinitis pigmentosa
   (viii) Adrenaline toxicity in aphakia
     (ix) Retinitis — *also: RP, Birdshot*
      (x) Vasculitis
     (xi) Irvine-Gass syndrome
    c. Choroid
       (i) Tumours, especially haemangioma
      (ii) Subretinal neovascularization
     (iii) Longstanding uveitis *pos plants!*

Irvine-Gass syndrome
1. Cystoid macular oedema occuring after cataract surgery
2. Occurs especially after intracapsular extraction with vitreous loss
3. 10–15% of cases are clinically evident
4. Detectable in 90% of cases with angiography
5. Most resolve by 6 months
6. Non-steroidal, anti-inflammatory drugs may help

Macular hole
1. Features
   a. Full thickness retinal hole
   b. Punched out lesion, usually ¼ disc diameter
   c. Round or oval
   d. Yellow pigment in floor may represent xanthophyll in macrophages
   e. Halo of oedema in surrounding retina
2. Causes
   a. Senile — from atrophic retina. Does not predispose to retinal detachment
   b. Trauma — due to vitreous traction or longstanding commotio retinae
   c. Myopia — often eyes with posterior staphylomas. Can cause retinal detachments
   d. Solar burns — small lamellar hole or cyst developing 2 weeks after exposure
   e. Severe chorioretinitis — following cystoid macular oedema.
3. Differential diagnosis
   a. Pseudomacular hole — gap in epiretinal membrane
   b. Lamellar hole — rupture of cyst in chronic macular oedema

Vitreoretinal interface maculopathy
Proliferation of epiretinal membranes. Contraction produces macular traction.
1. Types
   a. Early (Cellophaning)
      (i) Often no visual symptoms
      (ii) Translucent sheen
      (iii) Retinal striae
      (iv) Slight retinal traction
   b. Late (Macular pucker)
      (i) Increasing distortion
      (ii) Opaque membrane visible
      (iii) Macular oedema
2. Causes
   a. Idiopathic
   b. Retinal detachment surgery (7% of cases)

   c. Photocoagulation (especially excessive panretinal
      photocoagulation)
   d. Cryotherapy (not as common as photocoagulation)
   e. Central or branch retinal vein occlusion
   f. Diabetic retinopathy
   g. Trauma
   h. Longstanding chorioretinitis
3. Treatment
   a. Conservative
   b. Surgical
     (i) Membrane peeling
     (ii) Useful if vision better than 6/18 and history short
     (iii) Full visual recovery uncommon

Choroidal folds
1. Features
   a. Horizontal parallel folds at posterior pole
   b. Alternating dark and light lines
   c. Fluorescein angiography shows hyperfluorescent crests and
      hypofluorescent troughs
2. Causes
   a. Idiopathic (associated with hypermetropia)
   b. Orbital disease
     (i) Dysthyroid eye disease
     (ii) Orbital cellulitis
     (iii) Orbital tumours
   c. Ocular disease
     (i) Scleral buckling procedures
     (ii) Scleritis
     (iii) Choroidal tumours
     (iv) Ocular hypotony
     (v) Ocular trauma
     (vi) Papilloedema

Drug-induced macular disease
— Red scotoma paracentral — 1st
1. Chloroquine
Follow q 6 mths —
   a. Uses
later → scotoma, ↓VA, blurred —
     (i) Malaria prophylaxis
early
     (ii) Rheumatoid arthritis
     (iii) Systemic lupus erythematosus
   b. Toxicity
     (i) Very few cases with a total dose of less than 300 g
       (250 mg daily for about 3 years)
     (ii) Ocular toxicity very unlikely with doses of less than
       4 mg/kg/day
     (iii) Drug binds to melanin and interacts with nucleic acids
   c. Ocular features
     (i) Reversible cornea verticillata *— not related to Bull's eye.*

    (ii) Premaculopathy — reversible
                            ✳ — scotoma to red targets between 4 and 9° from fixation
    (iii) Maculopathy — irreversible
                      — may worsen despite withdrawal of drug
                      — visual impairment
                      — central scotoma *white*.
                      — central hyperpigmentation with hypopigmented surround (Bull's eye)
                      — EOG reduced

2. Hydroxychloroquine
  a. Lower incidence of retinal toxicity than chloroquine
  b. Toxicity
    (i) Toxicity unlikely if cumulative dose does not exceed 200 g (a maximum dose of 600 mg daily is equivalent to 219 g in one year)
    (ii) Toxicity very unlikely with doses of less than 6.5 mg/kg/day
3. Chlorpromazine
  a. Major tranquillizer
  b. Rarely causes RPE damage
  c. Toxicity at doses of 2.4 g daily over several years
4. Thioridazine
  a. Major tranquillizer
  b. Ocular features
    (i) Retinal pigment clumping and plaques
    (ii) Secondary RPE and choriocapillaris atrophy
  c. Toxicity unlikely at doses of 800 mg per day
5. Tamoxifen
  a. Anti-oestrogen used in the treatment of carcinoma of the breast
  b. Ocular features
    (i) Cystoid macular oedema
    (ii) RPE atrophy
    (iii) Intraretinal opacities

Causes of a bull's eye maculopathy
1. Chloroquine retinopathy
2. Hydroxychloroquine retinopathy
3. Cone dystrophy
4. Batten's disease
5. Benign concentric annular macular dystrophy

Hereditary disorders of the retina and choroid

Hereditary disorders of the retina and choroid account for 33% of the blind in developed countries and 70–90% of blind children

INVESTIGATIONS OF HEREDITARY RETINAL AND CHOROIDAL DISEASES

1. Visual acuity assessment
2. Colour vision testing
   a. Pseudoisochromatic plates
   b. Farnsworth-Munsell 100 hue test
   c. City university colour plates
   d. Nagel anomaloscope
   e. D15 test
3. Adaptometry — measurement of threshold stimulus change with time following retinal bleaching using Goldmann adaptometer
4. Fluorescein angiography
5. Electrodiagnostic tests
6. Biochemical studies in metabolic disease
7. Genetic studies
   a. Chromosome morphology
   b. Genetic markers
   c. Disease locus linkage studies using restriction fragment length polymorphism (RFLP)
   d. Biochemical products of abnormal genes
8. Screening
   a. Family tree
   b. Detection of carriers
9. Prenatal diagnosis
   a. Amniocentesis
   b. Fetoscopy
   c. Ultrasonography
   d. Chorionic villous sampling

Electro-oculogram (EOG)
1. Indirect measurement of standing potential of eye (6 mV)
2. Uses standardized ocular movements (30° excursion every 12 seconds for 12 minutes)
3. Potential originates in RPE
4. Potential changes with adaptive state
5. Arden index = $\dfrac{\text{highest potential in photopic state (light peak)}}{\text{lowest potential in scotopic state (dark trough)}}$

   Normal: > 1.85

Electroretinogram (ERG)
1. Recording of potentials in retina under the influence of light
2. Features
   a. Early receptor potential (ERP). Positive deflection originating from outer segment of photoreceptors. Response to intense stimulus. Potential proportional to stimulus intensity
   b. a wave. Negative deflection originating from inner segment of photoreceptors increasing with stimulus to maximum
   c. b wave. Positive deflection. Origin Müller's cells. Biphasic in mesopic conditions. b_1 = cone response, b_2 = rod response
   d. Oscillatory potentials. Small deflections on b wave. Origin bipolar cells
   e. c wave. Positive deflection originating in RPE
3. Types (to differentiate retinal components)
   a. Flicker. Rod ERG. Low frequency, low luminance stimuli. Dark adapted eye
      Cone ERG. Frequency > 15/min
   b. Dynamic. Suppressing rod function with pretest bleaching
   c. Static.   Rods. Scotopic conditions
      Cones. Photoptic conditions
   d. Pattern. Response to changing pattern stimuli. Small amplitude (2 mV). Originating mainly in ganglion cells

Visually evoked potentials (VEPs)
1. Averaged recording of visual cortex activity in response to light stimulus
2. Latency — 90–114 ms
3. Amplitude — approximately 10 mV
4. Types
   a. Flash. Response representing function of central 20° of retina
   b. Pattern. Response representing function of fovea. Response increases with pattern size reduction (60° to 15° subtended). Indication of visual acuity

Specific management aims in hereditary retinal/choroidal disease
1. Provision of prognosis
2. Specific treatments
3. Genetic counselling
4. Prenatal diagnosis and selective abortion
5. Referral to patient self-help groups

Hereditary malformations
1. Macular coloboma — occasionally autosomal dominant
2. Myelinated nerve fibres — symptomless, occasionally familial
   (AD, AR)
3. Posterior hyperplastic primary vitreous (AR)
   Features
   a. Retinal folds (especially inferiorly)
   b. Persistent hyaloid artery
   c. Cataract
   d. Vitreous bands
4. Norrie's disease (XLR)
   Features
   a. Impaired hearing
   b. Mental retardation
   c. Bilateral congenital blindness
   d. Bilateral retrolental vascular masses
   e. Cataract
   f. Phthisis
5. Incontinentia pigmenti (XL)
   Features
   a. Lethal to males
   b. Recurrent vesicobullous eruptions
   c. Cutaneous pigmentation
   d. Retrolental mass (dysplastic retina)
   e. Cataract
   f. Optic atrophy
   g. Nystagmus
   h. Squint

Vitreoretinal abnormalities
1. Juvenile schisis (XLR)
   Types
   a. Foveal
      (i) Late onset visual failure (over 20 years)
      (ii) Coalescing petaloid pattern of cystoid spaces in nerve
           fibre layer
      (iii) Late macular atrophy
      (iv) Associated with peripheral schisis (50%)
   b. Peripheral
      (i) May be present at birth
      (ii) 50% bilateral and inferotemporal

(iii) Splitting of nerve fibre layer
(iv) Vitreous veils, silver wiring, vitreous haemorrhage
(v) Retinal detachment rare (10%)
2. Wagner's disease (AD)
Features
a. Vitreous degeneration (veils)
b. Peripheral retinal degeneration (lattice)
c. Retinal vascular sclerosis
d. Myopia
e. Cataract (posterior subcapsular)
f. Retinal detachment
3. Stickler's syndrome (AD)   *more common than Marfans!!*
Features
a. Hereditary progressive arthro-ophthalmopathy
b. Marfanoid habitus
c. Vitreoretinal degeneration (similar to Wagner's) — *RDS, -ters.*
4. Goldmann-Favre disease (AR)   *-myopia*
Features   *(Pierre Robin → cleft palate*
a. Night blindness   *— Arthritis.)*
b. Foveal schisis
c. Pigmentary retinal degeneration
d. Cataract
e. Extinguished ERG

Disorders of photoreceptors
1. Congenital colour defects
Red and green defects — 8% of white males   } (XLR)
                       — 0.4% of females
Blue defects — tritanomaly (XLR)
             — tritanopia (AD)
Types
a. Anomalous trichomats
(i) Require abnormal mixtures of primary colours
(ii) Normal colour matches appear wrong
(iii) Defects — protanomalous (abnormal red)
             — deuteranomalous (abnormal green)
             — tritanomalous (abnormal blue)
b. Dichromats
(i) Require only two primary colours to match other colours
(ii) Accept normal colour matches
(iii) Defects — protanope (absent red)
             — deuteranope (absent green)
             — tritanope (absent blue)
2. Congenital achromatopsia (monochromatism)
a. Complete rod monochromatism (AR)
Features
(i) Complete absence of cones

      (ii) Photophobia, nystagmus
     (iii) Day blindness, defective colour vision
     (iv) Vision reduced (about 6/60 level)
      (v) Abnormal photoptic ERG
     (vi) Variants — incomplete (XLR)
                    — blue cone (XLR)
  b. Cone monochromatism (inheritance unknown)
    Features
      (i) Normal rods and only one cone type
     (ii) Colour blind
    (iii) Good vision
3. Night blindness (nyctalopia)
  a. Congenital nonprogressive nyctalopia (AD)
    Features
      (i) No macroscopic fundal pathology
     (ii) Monophasic adaptation
    (iii) Reduced scotopic b wave on ERG
    (iv) Possible defective neural transmission
  b. Nyctalopia with myopia (XLR)
    Features
      (i) Myopia (4–15 D)
     (ii) Poor vision (6/60)
  c. Oguchi disease (AR)
    Features
      (i) Occurs in Japanese
     (ii) Nyctalopia with slow adaptation
    (iii) Grey-white fundus appearing normal after period in
         dark (Mitzuo phenomenon)

Retinitis pigmentosa
1. Group of progressive disorders (Rod - cone dystr)
2. Triad of
  a. Night blindness
  b. Visual field defect
  c. Typical fundal appearance
3. Symptoms
  a. Night blindness
  b. Visual difficulty due to field loss
  c. Photophobia, glare
  d. Family history
  e. Associated defects
4. Signs
  a. Early
      (i) Reduced dark adaptation
     (ii) Annular scotoma
    (iii) Equatorial patchy RPE atrophy and hypertrophy
    (iv) Narrowing of retinal vessels

b. Late
   (i) Tubular fields (2–3°)
   (ii) Bone corpuscle pigmentation
   (iii) Choroidal atrophy
   (iv) Retinal venous sheathing
   (v) Drusen
   (vi) Waxy disc pallor

5. Associated findings
  a. Myopia
  b. Keratoconus
  c. Optic disc drusen
  d. Posterior subcapsular lens opacities
  e. Glaucoma
  f. Cystoid macular oedema

6. Investigations
  a. EOG. Lost early
  b. ERG. Progressive rod and cone loss

7. Inheritance — Varies depending on survey and country
  a. AR   51% — *worst*
  b. AD   26% - *best prognosis.*
  c. XLR   23%

8. Prognosis — 25% maintain adequate reading vision

9. Atypical variations
  a. Sine pigmento — inconspicuous pigmentary changes
  b. Macular type (AD, AR) — preceeding macular changes
  c. Pericentric/central (AR) — possible rod–cone dystrophy
  d. Sectoral (AD) — symmetrical, bilateral
                    — commonly inferonasal
                    — ERG reduced
  e. Unilateral — doubtful existence
  f. Progressive albipunctate dystrophy (AR, AD) — night
    —(Retinitis punctata albescense). blindness
                                     — field loss
                                     progressive
                                   — white dots
                                   in fundus
                                   — ERG
                                   reduced
  g. Fundus albipunctatus — congenital nonprogressive
                     nyctalopia
                     — widespread peripheral white dots
  h. Leber's congenital amaurosis (AD) — congenital severe
                               blindness (less than
                               6/60)
                     — ERG reduced
                     — associated with renal
                         abnormalities and
                         deafness

Variable fundal findings
  (i) Initially little change
  (ii) Salt and pepper fundus
  (iii) Late RP-like picture
  (iv) Optic atrophy
Associated ocular features
  (i) Nystagmus
  (ii) Oculo-digital syndrome
  (iii) Photophobia
  (iv) Cataract
  (v) Keratoconus
  (vi) Strabismus

Disorders associated with retinitis pigmentosa
1. Metabolic disorders
  a. Bassen-Kornzweig syndrome (AR)
    (i) Absence of beta-lipoprotein
    (ii) Features — early — steatorrhoea, acanthocytosis
        — late — ataxia, RP-like fundus
    (iii) Treatment — large doses of vitamin A and E
        — decrease intake of long chain fatty acids
        — improvement occurs
  b. Refsum's disease (AR)
    (i) Phytanic acid storage disease
    (ii) Features — hypertrophic peripheral neuropathy
        — ataxia
        — deafness
        — cardiomyopathy
        — icthyosis
    (iii) Treatment — eliminate phytates (dairy products)
  c. Batten's disease
  d. Gangliosidoses
  e. Mucopolysaccharidoses
2. Mitochondrial muscle dystrophy
  a. Results in a chronic progressive external ophthalmoplegia
  b. Kearns-Sayre syndrome
    (i) Progressive external ophthalmoplegia
    (ii) Pigmentary retinopathy
    (iii) Heart block due to cardiomyopathy
3. Dystrophia myotonica
4. Neurological disorders
  a. Ataxia
    (i) Friedreich's (AR)
    (ii) Marie's (AD)
  b. Deafness
    (i) Usher's syndrome (AR) — 5% of childhood deafness
        — cataracts may occur
    (ii) Hallgren's syndrome — deafness, ataxia, psychiatric

disturbances and presenile
cataract
(iii) Alstrom's syndrome — deafness, obesity, diabetes
mellitus, renal impairment,
baldness, acanthosis nigricans,
raised uric acid and
triglycerides, skeletal
abnormalities and
hypogonadism
(iv) Laurence–Moon–Bardet–Biedl syndrome (AR) —
deafness, polydactyly, mental retardation, obesity and
hypogonadism
(v) Cockayne's syndrome (AR) — deafness, cataract,
dwarfism, mental
retardation and progeria

Causes of pseudoretinitis pigmentosa
1. Infections
   a. Syphilis retinopathy
   b. Rubella retinopathy
2. Calcium oxalate retinopathy
3. Ocular injury
4. Spontaneous retinal reattachment
5. Drug-induced
   a. Quinine
   b. Phenothiazines
6. Vascular occlusion

Management of retinitis pigmentosa
1. Genetic counselling
2. Referral to self-help groups
3. Management of associated ocular findings, e.g. glaucoma and
   cataract
4. Exclude treatable metabolic disorders
5. Avoid excessive illumination, which may have a role in
   disease progression

Cone dystrophy (AD)
Types I
   a. Reduced photopic vision
   b. Photophobia
   c. Onset 10–30 years
   d. Bulls-eye macular appearance
   e. Photopic ERG abnormal
Type II
   a. More severe disease
   b. Extensive changes (bone spicule)

Sjögren's dystrophy (AR)
Features
    a. Childhood onset
    b. Vision normal initially
    c. Initial dark pigment spot in central macula
    d. Progressive pericentral pigmentation

Butterfly dystrophy (uncertain inheritance)
Butterfly-shaped central pigmentation

Sorsby's dystrophy (AD)
Features
    a. Bilateral
    b. Patients usually 30–50 years of age
    c. Retinal oedema, exudates and haemorrhage in macular area
    d. Progresses to choroidoretinal atrophy

Familial drusen (AD)
    1. Most common flecked macular syndrome
    2. Features
        a. Onset after 20 years
        b. Bilateral, central yellow lesions
        c. Electrodiagnostic tests normal

Stargardt's disease (AR)
    1. Features
        a. Central visual loss
        b. Onset 10–20 years
    2. Types
        a. Central
            Atrophic ovoid foveal (beaten bronze) lesion
        b Central and pericentral
            (i) Pigmentary retinopathy
            (ii) Fishtail lesions (white) at posterior pole
        c. Central and peripheral
            (i) Pigmentary retinopathy
            (ii) Vessel narrowing
            (iii) Disc pallor
            (iv) EOG slightly reduced
            (v) ERG progressive cone loss

Fundus flavimaculatus (AR) — variant of Stargardt's
Features
    a. Progressive, powdery, central fishtail lesions at RPE level
    b. 50% have Stargardt's-type fovea

Best's vitelliform dystrophy (AD)
1. Features
   a. Bilateral
   b. Variable appearance
   c. Average onset 6 years
   d. Abnormal EOG in carriers
2. Stages
   (i) Previtelliform — abnormal EOG
   (ii) Vitelliform — macular cyst composed of lipofuscin
   (iii) Pseudohypopyon — cyst absorption reducing colour vision
   (iv) Vitelliruptive — scrambled egg appearance, reduced vision
   (v) End stage — loss of vision due to
       — macular scarring
       — disciform degeneration
       — macular atrophy

CHOROIDAL DEGENERATIONS
1. Central areolar sclerosis (AR, AD)
   Features
       (i) Onset 20–40 years
       (ii) Bilateral central atrophy
       (iii) Progressive visual loss
       (iv) ERG and EOG are normal
2. Generalized choroidal atrophy (AD)
   — widespread choriocapillaris atrophy
3. Gyrate atrophy (AR)
   a. Deficiency of ornithine ketoacid aminotransferase
   b. Features
       (i) Onset 10–30 years
       (ii) Night blindness, tunnel vision
       (iii) Patchy, coalescing, progressive, equatorial choroidal atrophy
       (iv) Myopia
       (v) Cataract
       (vi) Reduced ERG and EOG
   c. Treatment
       (i) High dose Vitamin B_6
       (ii) Proline supplementation
4. Choroideremia (XLR)
   a. Features
       (i) Onset 5–10 years
       (ii) Night blindness progressing to blindness
   b. Fundal findings
       (i) Early — granular pigmentary changes
       (ii) Late — total choroidal atrophy

    c. Carrier state — mid peripheral pigmentary changes which do not progress

5. Degenerative myopia
    a. Seventh commonest cause of blind registration in UK
    b. Blindness often results in young adulthood
    c. Features
        (i) Cornea — increased corneal diameter
        (ii) Trabecular meshwork — chronic open angle glaucoma
                                      — steroid responsiveness
        (iii) Lens — posterior subcapsular opacities
        (iv) Vitreous — syneresis and synchysis
                       — posterior detachment
                       — opacities
        (v) Retina— straightening of retinal vessels
                    — macular hole
                    — peripheral retinal holes and degenerations, e.g. lattice
        (vi) Choroid/RPE — pallor
                       — tessellation
                       — hyperpigmentation at macula
                       — lacquer cracks (yellow-white lines representing cracks in Bruch's membrane; 4% of high myopes)
                       — Subretinal neovascularization at the macula
                       — Foster-Fuch's spot. Elevated and varying in colour
        (vii) Choroid/sclera — posterior staphyloma
        (viii) Optic disc — pallor
                       — enlargement, usually due to optical magnification
                       — crescents, may encircle the disc, but more commonly temporal. White (scleral). Pigmented (choroidal)
                       — central retinal artery and vein bifurcating on (usually temporal) disc surface (T-sign)

STORAGE DISORDERS ASSOCIATED WITH FUNDAL PATHOLOGY

1. Sphingolipidoses
    a. Tay-Sachs disease (AR)
        Features — normal at birth
                   — fatal by 3 years
                   — hypotonia, hyperacusis, convulsions

         — cherry-red macular spot (early)
         — reduced VER
         — serum hexosaminadase-A level diagnostic
         — ganglion cells laden with membranous
           cytoplasmic bodies

  b. Sandhoff's disease (AR)
     Features — similar to Tay-Sachs
            — extensive visceral involvement

  c. Sulphated cerebrosidosis (AR)
    (i) Group of diseases
   (ii) Features — infantile onset
              — ataxia
              — mental retardation
              — grey perifoveal infiltrate
              — fatal disorder

  d. Niemann–Pick disease (AR)
    (i) Group of disorders. Most important form is Group A
       (infantile)
   (ii) Features — hepatosplenomegaly
              — retarded physical and mental development
              — cherry-red macular spot
              — late optic atrophy
              — foam cells in bone marrow biopsy

2. Batten's disease (AR)
  a. Accumulation of autofluorescent lipopigments in neural,
    visceral and somatic tissues
  b. Most important form is juvenile (onset 4–6 years)
  c. Features — psychomotor deterioration
            — visual failure
            — increasing white macular spot
            — vessel narrowing
            — optic atrophy
            — pigmentary disturbance
            — vacuolated lymphocytes and abnormal
              peroxidase activity in blood
            — ceroid bodies in skeletal muscle, white blood
              cells, Schwann cells, rectal, skin and
              conjunctival tissue

3. Cherry-red spot — myoclonus syndrome (AR)
  Features — myoclonic siezures
          — normal intelligence
          — cherry-red spot (early)
          — deteriorating vision
          — ERG normal
          — VEP reduced

4. Mucopolysaccharidoses (AR)
  a. Extensive accumulation of MPS
  b. 6 types, distinguished by urinalysis

    c. Features — corneal clouding
                — optic atrophy
                — mental retardation
                — physical deformity
    d. Types associated with pigmentary retinopathy
       (i) MPS 1H — Hurler's syndrome
      (ii) MPS 1S — Scheie's syndrome
     (iii) MPS 2 — Hunter's syndrome
     (iv) MPS 3 — Sanfilippo's syndrome

ALBINISM

1. Failure of melanocyte or melanosome system in varying amounts, producing varying deficiency of melanin
2. Biochemistry

Phenylalanine $\longrightarrow$ Tyrosine $\underset{a}{\longrightarrow}$ Dihydroxyphenylalanine (DOPA) $\downarrow b$

                                          Melanin

Enzyme defects
a. Tyrosinase negative albinism
b. Tyrosinase positive albinism

Types of albinism
1. Generalized type oculocutaneous (AR)
    a. Tyrosinase positive group
       (i) Differentiated by hair bulb incubation in tyrosine solution (producing pigmentation) after age 4 years
      (ii) Features — mild, improving with age
                    — iris transillumination
                    — nystagmus
                    — poor vision
                    — refractive errors
    b. Tyrosinase negative group
       Features — severe disease
                  — photophobic
                  — poor vision
                  — nystagmus
                  — iris transillumination
                  — no fundal pigmentation
                  — absent foveal reflex
                  — refractive errors
                  — 90% of fibres decussate at chiasm
                  — lateral geniculate body organization abnormal
                  — negative hair bulb test
    c. Yellow mutant group
       Features — normal skin pigmentation develops
                  — ocular changes persist

    d. Hermansky–Pudlak syndrome   *Puerto Rican*:
       (i) Sub-group of tyrosinase negative
      (ii) Associated haemorrhagic diathesis
     (iii) Avoid drugs blocking prostaglandin synthetase
    e. Chédiak-Higashi syndrome
       (i) Features   — mild albinism
                     — altered immunity, recurrent infections
                     — fatal disease
                     — neutrophils show large inclusion bodies
                     — total lack of RPE pigmentation
      (ii) Treatment — vitamin C may improve leucocyte function
  2. Ocular type (XLR)
    a. Confined to eyes
    b. Abnormality of optic cup derived melanocytes
    c. Giant melanosomes in RPE
    d. Carriers
       (i) Iris transillumination
      (ii) RPE granularity
  3. Partial type (AD)
    a. Albinoid features
    b. Eyes not affected

Ocular tumours

IRIS NAEVUS

1. Slightly elevated discrete pigmented mass
2. Benign, usually spindle A or B cell type
3. Serial observation required

CHOROIDAL NAEVUS

1. 10% of adult caucasians
2. Flat or slightly elevated
3. Oval with indistinct margins with or without overlying drusen
4. Occasionally associated with disciform macular degeneration

Rx Observe - 5% grow in 1 year. have VF defects.

MALIGNANT MELANOMA OF IRIS

1. Features
   a. Average age 40–50 years
   b. Ectropion uveae
   c. Pupillary distortion
   d. Neovascularization
   e. Local lens opacities
   f. Secondary glaucoma
   g. Uveitis
2. Types
   a. Nodular   ⎫ Pigmented or amelanotic
   b. Diffuse   ⎬ Usually spindle A or B
3. Treatment
   a. Observation
   b. Local resection

MALIGNANT MELANOMA OF CILIARY BODY

1. 15% of uveal melanomas
2. Features
   a. Late presentation
   b. Lens subluxation

    c. Uveitis
    d. Secondary glaucoma
    e. Sentinel episcleral vessels
    f. Failure of accommodation
  3. Types
    a. Localized
    b. Diffuse or annular (poor prognosis) ←

MALIGNANT MELANOMA OF CHOROID

  1. Features
    a. Average age 50–60 years
    b. Rare in non-whites
    c. May arise in pre-existing naevus
    d. May contain orange pigmentation (lipofuscin)
    e. Presentation
      (i) Visual field loss
     (ii) Macular involvement
    (iii) Serous retinal detachment
    (iv) Uveitis
     (v) Secondary glaucoma *by NVI or cells.*
    (vi) Chance finding
  2. Types
    a. Localized
    b. Diffuse (rare, poor prognosis)
    c. Pigmented or amelanotic
  3. Spread
    a. Local
    b. Haematogenous (especially to liver)
  4. Histology *Callender classification*
    a. Cellular type
      (i) Spindle A — spindle-shaped cells, flattened nucleus, no nucleoli
     (ii) Spindle B — round/oval nucleus, prominent nucleoli
    (iii) Epithelioid — large oval/round cells, eosinophilic cytoplasm, round nuclei, prominent nucleoli, many mitotic figures
    b. Histological features
      (i) Fascicular — palisading of cells
     (ii) Mixed — spindle and epithelioid cells
    (iii) Necrotic — cell type not recognizable
  5. Features which indicate a poor prognosis
    a. Large size
    b. Extraocular spread
    c. Presence of epithelioid cells and necrosis
    d. Anteriorly placed tumour
    e. Diffuse tumour
    f. Rupture of Bruch's membrane

extraocular

Dx u/s, CT/MRI, P³², *Transillumination, Indirect, contact lens, * IVFA Photos (baseline).

    g. Increasing age

    h. Near optic disc

6. Differential diagnosis
   a. Benign naevus
   b. Metastatic carcinoma
   c. Pigment epithelial hyperplasia
   d. Retinal detachment
   e. Choroidal haemangioma
   f. Disciform degeneration
   g. Congenital ciliary body cyst
   h. Melanocytoma
   i. Astrocytoma
   j. Choroidal haemorrhage/detachment

7. Management — controversial; tailored to patient's requirements
   a. Observation *— small or elderly, or mets —*
   b. General examination (to exclude metastases) *CT liver*
   c. Enucleation *— large, or blind eye*
   d. Photocoagulation *— v.y. small tumors* *→ Proton beam good future.*
   e. Irradiation, e.g. local plaque, charged particle beam
   f. Local resection *→ small <3 mm — 10 Diam*
   g. Cryotherapy *> Peripheral > medium <3-5 mm — 10-15 D/mm*
   h. Exenteration *height.*
   i. Palliation *— chemo.* *★ I¹²⁵, Co⁶⁰*
   — immuno.

Key ★ ☆

METASTATIC DEPOSITS

Commonest intraocular tumours

1. Features
   a. Often multiple
   b. White, round lesions
   c. Respond to local radiotherapy
2. Primary source
   a. Breast ♀
   b. Lung ♂⁺
   c. Gastrointestinal tract
   d. Kidney
   e. Prostate
   f. Thyroid
   g. Testes

Other tumours

1. Haemangioma of iris
2. Choroidal haemangiomas
   a. Localized
      (i) Red–orange lesion
      (ii) RPE mottling and atrophy
      (iii) Serous detachment

b. Diffuse
 — Associated with Sturge-Weber syndrome
3. Juvenile xanthogranuloma
 a. Yellow–orange accumulations in iris *Touton Giant cells!!
 b. May present with spontaneous hyphaema   VCT for bone D's
4. Choroidal osteoma – young ♀   of *histiocytosis X.
 a. Rare
 b. Bone formation

TUMOURS OF CILIARY BODY EPITHELIUM

1. Congenital ciliary body cysts
2. Fuchs' adenoma (benign)
3. Medulloepithelioma
 a. Rare tumour of ciliary epithelium
 b. Benign or malignant
 c. Children (average age 5 years)
 d. Usually locally invasive

RETINAL ASTROCYTOMA

1. Benign
2. Associated with tuberose sclerosis
3. 15% bilateral
4. Single or multiple slow growing tumours at or near optic disc
5. Usually nodular
6. Translucent, late calcification (mulberry tumour)

RETINAL CAPILLARY HAEMANGIOMAS

1. Features
 a. Associated with von Hippel-Lindau disease
 b. Average age 20–30 years
 c. Gradually enlarging orange–red tumour
 d. Feeder artery and draining vein
 e. Leaking vessels produce
  (i) Retinal exudates
  (ii) Serous retinal detachment
  (iii) Retinal haemorrhage
2. Treatment
 a. Early detection in at risk patients
 b. Photocoagulation
 c. Cryotherapy

RETINAL CAVERNOUS HAEMANGIOMA

1. Congenital
2. Unilateral
3. Aneurysmal lesions with 'cluster of grapes' appearance in inner retina or optic nerve head
4. Asymptomatic

RETINAL RACEMOSE HAEMANGIOMA

1. Congenital unilateral arteriovenous malformation
2. Enlarged tortuous vessels
3. Affects retina or optic nerve head
4. Associated with Wyburn-Mason syndrome

RETINOBLASTOMA

1. Features
   a. Tumour of primitive photoreceptor cells
   b. Commonest childhood ocular malignancy of eye
   c. Average age at presentation is 18 months
   d. Prevalence = 1:20 000, Males = Females
   e. Increased risk of other tumours especially osteosarcoma
2. Inheritance
   a. Up to 40% hereditary
   b. Retinoblastoma gene located on the long arm of chromosome 13 close to esterase D gene. Levels of esterase D can be used as a genetic marker in some cases
   c. Increased incidence with Trisomy 13, 21, and deletion of long arm of 13
   d. Bilateral cases always inherited
   e. Increased risk with increasing paternal age
3. Presentation
   a. Leukocoria
   b. Strabismus
   c. Secondary glaucoma
   d. Proptosis (especially developing countries)
   e. Anterior uveitis, hyphaema, pseudohypopyon
   f. Routine examination
4. Appearance
   a. Endophytic — within vitreous cavity. White/pinkish nodular lesion with surface vessels
   b. Exophytic — growing in subretinal space, usually with retinal detachment
5. Differential diagnosis
   a. Retinopathy of prematurity
   b. Persistent primary hyperplastic vitreous ← *microphthalmic eye!! Never in RB ciliary processes.*

    c. Congenital cataract
    d. Toxocara/toxoplasma ~ ELIZA test.
    e. Retinal astrocytoma
    f. Retinal dysplasia ~ also rosettes
    g. Coats' disease
    h. Medulloepithelioma ~ cousin of Rb! see rosettes.
    i. Retinal angiomas
    j. Coloboma
    k. Retinal detachment
    l. Norrie's disease

6. Histopathology
    a. Small closely packed polygonal cells
    b. High nuclear/cytoplasmic ratio
    c. Attempted differentiation produces Flexner-Wintersteiner only RB! rosettes
    d. Necrosis may produce pseudorosettes
    e. Calcification can occur

Homer wright → (medulloblastoma Neuroblastoma).

7. Spread
    a. Trans-sclerally into orbit
    b. Direct along optic nerve
    c. Via subarachnoid space to CNS
    d. Haematogenous, to bone marrow

8. Features which indicate a poor prognosis
    a. Metastatic spread
    b. Invasion of orbit or sclera
    c. Extension to resected end of optic nerve
    d. Large tumour
    e. Intraocular complications, e.g. cataract, rubeosis and pseudohypopyon
    f. Poor cellular differentiation with lack of rosettes
    g. Vitreous seeding

9. Diagnosis (N.B. Biopsy contraindicated)
    a. History and ocular/general examination
    b. Family history and examination of relatives
    c. Imaging — ultrasound, radiography and CT scan (Look for calcification)
    d. Biochemistry
       (i) Alpha-fetoprotein and carcinoembryonic antigen
       (ii) Aqueous/blood lactate dehydrogenase ratio
       (iii) Esterase D levels
    e. Serology — toxocara/toxoplasma titres
    f. Gene probes

10. Management
    a. Of patient
       (i) Ocular examination (bilateral or unilateral)
       (ii) General examination to exclude metastases
         — Unilateral. Enucleation if large

— Bilateral. Radiation – *Extnl Beam* >> *plaque*
Cryotherapy ×3 *per month*
Photocoagulation
— Metastatic. Systemic chemotherapy
  (iii) Regular follow up in early years
b. Of family
  (i) Genetic counselling
  (ii) Ocular examination of near relatives

Ocular motility

THE EXTRAOCULAR MUSCLES

1. Features
   a. Highly specialized striated muscles
   b. Small fibres peripherally
      (i) slow twitch
      (ii) multiple motor end plates ('en grappe')
      (iii) graded contractions in absence of action potential
   c. Large fibres centrally
      (i) fast twitch
      (ii) single motor end plate
   d. Small motor unit. 1 axon supplies 6 muscle fibres
   e. Proprioception via 5th nerve (mesencephalic nucleus)
   f. Specialized muscle spindles
2. The Recti
   a. All have origin from annulus of Zinn
   b. 4 cm long
   c. Scleral insertions
      (i) medial rectus (MR) 5.5 mm from limbus
      (ii) inferior rectus (IR) 6.5 mm from limbus
      (iii) lateral rectus (LR) 7.0 mm from limbus
      (iv) superior rectus (SR) 7.5 mm from limbus
   d. Tendon length
      (i) MR 4.0 mm
      (ii) IR 5.5 mm
      (iii) LR 9.0 mm
      (iv) SR 5.8 mm
   e. Insertion width
      (i) MR 10.3 mm
      (ii) IR 9.8 mm
      (iii) LR 9.2 mm
      (iv) SR 10.6 mm
   f. In the primary position of gaze the SR and IR form an angle of 22.5° with the ocular axis
   g. Nerve supply
      (i) MR and IR — inferior division of 3rd

(ii) SR — superior division of 3rd
(iii) LR — 6th
3. Superior oblique (SO)
   a. Origin from lesser wing of sphenoid superomedial to annulus of Zinn
   b. Passes anteriorly above MR
   c. 6 cm long (3 cm muscle, 3 cm tendon)
   d. Passes through trochlea 4 cm from origin
   e. 11 mm width insertion behind equator in superotemporal quadrant of globe passing beneath SR
   f. In the primary position of gaze it forms an angle of 51° with the ocular axis
   g. Supplied, on its upper surface, by 4th
4. Inferior oblique (IO)
   a. Origin from orbital floor (vertically below trochlea)
   a. Passes obliquely backwards inferior to IR
   c. Covered laterally by LR at insertion
   d. 3.7 cm long
   e. In the primary position of gaze it forms an angle of 51° with the ocular axis
   f. 9 mm width insertion behind the equator, 2 mm below and lateral to the macula
   g. Supplied by the inferior division of 3rd

Table 5

Muscle actions	Primary	Secondary
Medial rectus	Adduction	—
Lateral rectus	Abduction	—
Superior rectus	Elevation (maximal in abduction)	Adduction, intorsion (maximal in adduction)
Inferior rectus	Depression (maximal in abduction)	Adduction, extorsion (maximal in adduction)
Superior oblique	Depression (maximal in adduction)	Abduction, intorsion (maximal in abduction)
Inferior oblique	Elevation (maximal in adduction)	Abduction, extorsion (maximal in abduction)

Eye movements

1. Ductions — monocular eye movements
   a. Adduction
   b. Abduction

    c. Elevation
    d. Depression
    e. Intorsion
    f. Extorsion
2. Versions — binocular eye movements in which the two eyes move synchronously and symmetrically in the same direction
    a. Dextroversion
    b. Laevoversion
    c. Upgaze
    d. Downgaze
    e. Dextroelevation
    f. Laevoelevation
    g. Dextrodepression
    h. Laevodepression
    i. Dextrocycloversion
    j. Laevocycloversion
3. Vergences — binocular movements in which both eyes move synchronously and symmetrically in opposite directions
    a. Convergence
       (i) Voluntary
      (ii) Reflex — tonic
                — proximal
                — fusional
                — accommodative
    b. Divergence
       (i) Voluntary
      (ii) Reflex (fusional)

AC/A ratio
Accommodative convergence exerted in response to one unit of accommodation (normally 3–5 : 1)
Measured by
1. Heterophoria method — prism cover test (PCT) at 6 m and 33 cm
2. Gradient method — PCT at 6 m then concave lenses inserted in trial frames (up to − 3 D) and PCT repeated

Yoke muscles
Muscle pairs acting in each of 6 cardinal positions, e.g.
Dextroelevation: right SR and left IO

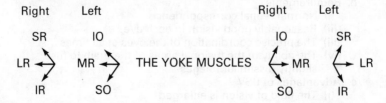

Sherrington's law of reciprocal innervation
Increase in innervation and contraction of a muscle is associated
with a reciprocal decrease in innervation of the antagonist

Hering's law of equal innervation
During any conjugate eye movement, equal and simultaneous
innervation flows to the yoke muscles

Hess Chart
Shows the position of the non-fixing eye in all positions of gaze
when the other eye is fixing. Based on
1. Foveal projection
2. Hering's and Sherrington's laws
3. Dissociation of the eyes using complementary colours or a
   mirror

Schematic representation of Hess chart

Field of 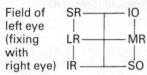  Field of
left eye   right
(fixing   eye
with   (fixing
right eye)   with
                                               left eye)

BINOCULAR FUNCTION
1. Binocular single vision (BSV) — the simultaneous use of the
   two eyes to give a single mental impression in normal
   conditions of seeing. Acquired and reinforced in the first three
   years of life
   a. Worth's classification
      Grade 1 = simultaneous perception
        (i) Paramacular
       (ii) Macular
      (iii) Foveal
      Grade 2 = fusion
        (i) Sensory (the ability to fuse two similar images)
       (ii) Motor, i.e. vergence
      Grade 3 = stereopsis
   b. Requirements
        (i) Normal retinal correspondence
       (ii) Reasonably good vision in each eye
      (iii) The precise coordination of the eyes at all times
       (iv) The ability of the fusional areas of the brain to fuse
            slightly dissimilar images
   c. Advantages of BSV
        (i) The field of vision is enlarged
       (ii) Elimination of the blind spot

     (iii) Binocular visual acuity is slightly greater than
          monocular
     (iv) Stereopsis allows very accurate depth perception
2. Horopter — an imaginary surface in space all points of which
    stimulate corresponding retinal points and are therefore
    projected to the same locus in space
3. Panum's space — that region around and including the
    horopter in which BSV can be obtained

Investigation of binocular function

Requires the assessment of the presence or absence of
1. Retinal correspondence (normal or abnormal)
2. Suppression
3. Fusion
4. Stereopsis

1. Assessment of retinal correspondence
   a. Bagolini glasses
   b. Major amblyoscope
   c. Lang's 2 pencil test
   d. Prism adaptation test
   e. Worth's 4 lights test
   f. Bagolini filter bar
   g. After image test
   h. Binocular visuoscopy
2. Assessment of suppression
   a. Diplopia tests for peripheral suppression, e.g. Worth's 4
      lights test
   b. Major amblyoscope (for peripheral suppression)
   c. 4 dioptre, prism test (for central suppression)
3. Assessment of fusion

Table 6 Normal amplitudes of fusion

	Near (Prism dioptres)	Distance (Prism dioptres)	Measure with
Convergence	35/40	15	Base out prism
Divergence	15	5	Base in prism
Vertical			
a. Supravergence	3	3	Base down prism
b. Infravergence	3	3	Base up prism
Total	6	6	
Cyclovergence (torsional)	(degrees)	(degrees)	
a. Incyclo	3	3	Major
b. Excyclo	3	3	amblyoscope
Total	6	6	

4. Assessment of stereopsis
    a. Qualitative tests
        (i) Lang's 2 pencil test
        (ii) Major amblyoscope
    b. Quantative tests
        (i) Titmus test
        (ii) TNO test
        (iii) Lang stereo test
        (iv) Frisby test
        (v) Randot test

AMBLYOPIA

Defective visual acuity which persists after correction of any
refractive error and removal of any pathological obstacle to vision
1. Classification
    a. Stimulus deprivation amblyopia (unilateral or bilateral,
        complete or partial)a .ex anopia'
    b. Strabismic
    c. Anisometropic
    d. Ametropic (high bilateral refractive error)
2. Treatment
    a. Occlusion (total or partial)
    b. Optical penalization
    c. Cycloplegic drugs

ASSESSMENT OF VISUAL ACUITY

1. Neonates
    a. Follow a light, face, object (ask mother)
    b. Optokinetic nystagmus
    c. Forced choice preferential looking
    d. Visually evoked potential
2. 3–6 months
    a. Visually directed reaching
    b. Catford drum
3. 6–18 months
    a. Worth's static balls
    b. Worth's rolling balls
    c. 'Hundreds and thousands' pick up test (approximates to
        6/24 vision at 33 cm)
4. 18 months–3 years
    a. Beale–Collins' pictures
    b. Ffookes symbols
    c. STYCAR 5 letter test (Screening Tests for Young Children
        And Retards)
5. 3–5 years (and illiterates)
    a. Sheridan–Gardiner test

b. E-test
c. Sjögren hand test
d. Landolt's broken rings
6. Literate children and adults
 a. Snellen chart (linear or single optotypes)
 b. Reading types
  (i) Reduced Snellen
  (ii) N (near) test
  (iii) J (Jaeger) test
  (iv) Maclure's reading books (for children)
  (v) Moorfields' bar reading book
  (vi) Merrick's reading book

ASSESSMENT OF OCULAR DEVIATION

1. Horizontal and vertical deviations
 a. Estimation
  (i) Cover test
  (ii) Hirschberg's method
  (iii) Krimsky prism reflection test
 b. Measurement
  (i) Prism cover test (BO for eso, BI for exo, BD for hypertropia)
  (ii) Major amblyoscope
  (iii) Maddox rod (for distance)
  (iv) Maddox wing (for near — 33 cm)
2. Torsion
 Measurement
  (i) 2 Maddox rods
  (ii) Away's cyclo test

NON-PARALYTIC STRABISMUS — ESOTROPIA

Classification
1. Primary Esotropia
 a. Non-accommodative
  (i) Constant — congenital (infantile) esotropia
   — nystagmus blockage syndrome
   — late onset esotropia
   — myopia associated esotropia
  (ii) Intermittent — convergence excess (near esotropia)
   — divergence insufficiency (distance esotropia)
   — cyclic esotropia
 b. Accommodative
  (i) Constant — partially accommodative esotropia
  (ii) Intermittent — fully accommodative esotropia (refractive)

*[handwritten margin notes]: Always check fundus * R/O RB!!! 2nd to R/O RB; 2nd cause of RB is strabismus; cyclic esotropia — becomes like — becomes constant, 24° cycle*

      (iii) Intermittent — accommodative esotropia with
               convergence excess (non-refractive)
2. Consecutive esotropia
  a. Features
    (i) Usually after surgical correction of primary exotropia
    (ii) Rarely spontaneous
  b. Management
    (i) If good BSV, surgery early
    (ii) If cosmetic, surgery as required
3. Secondary (symptomatic) esotropia
  a. Features
    (i) When there is severe visual loss in one eye or
       asymmetrical visual loss
    (ii) If congenital or infantile loss, eye may converge or
       diverge
    (iii) If childhood loss, usually converge
    (iv) If adult loss, usually diverge
  b. Management
    (i) Correct visual loss
    (ii) Surgery for cosmesis

Congenital (infantile) esotropia
1. Features
  a. Onset in first six months of life
  b. Large constant angle
  c. Crossed fixation
  d. Alternating or preference
  e. Compensatory head posture (CHP)
  f. Amblyopia infrequent
  g. Emmetropic or low hypermetropia
  h. Dissociated vertical deviation (DVD)
  i. Latent nystagmus
  j. Bilateral inferior oblique overaction (in 20%)
  k. Increased incidence of developmental and neurological
    abnormalities
2. Management
  a. Correct any significant ametropia and treat any amblyopia
  b. Surgery

Late onset esotropia
1. Features
  a. Constant eso with onset at 2–4 years
  b. Large angle
  c. Diplopia usually present (especially early)
  d. Little or no refractive error
  e. Normal retinal correspondence and fusion
2. Management — surgery

Non-accommodative convergence excess esotropia
1. Features   N > D.
    a. Intermittent
    b. Controlled for distance, manifest for near
    c. AC/A ratio normal
    d. Emmetropia or low hypermetropia
2. Management
    a. Correct ametropia
    b. Surgery

Non-accommodative divergence insufficiency
1. Features   D > N
    a. Intermittent
    b. Manifest for distance, controlled for near
    c. No amblyopia
    d. Emmetropia
2. Management
    a. Try BO prisms if small angle
    b. Surgery rarely .   Div. paralysis → pontine
                                                            tumor.

Partially accommodative esotropia   combined - Accom c AC/A
1. Features
    a. Hypermetropic
    b. Onset age 1–3 years
    c. Deviation greater for near fixation (N > D) high AC/A.
    d. Constant deviation reduced but not eliminated by
       hypermetropic correction
    e. More commonly unilateral
    f. Inferior oblique overaction is common
    g. Amblyopia common
2. Management
    a. Correct the refractive error , Try bifocals but usually needs
    b. Treat amblyopia   surgery for remaining
    c. Assess BSV   eso. !
    d. Surgery

Fully accommodative esotropia   NL AC/A
1. Features
    a. Moderate hypermetropia   3-10
    b. BSV usually present
    c. Occasional microtropia
    d. Onset at 2–5 years often after febrile illness
    e. Intermittent, seen when tired or unwell
    f. Correction of hypermetropia usually eliminates deviation 3° 10°
    g. Deviation approximately equal for near and distance (N = D)
    h. AC/A ratio normal
    i. Amblyopia rare

2. Management
    a. Full correction of hypermetropia — *leave esophoria* -
    b. Occlusion if necessary
    c. Orthoptic exercises
        (i) Diplopia recognition
        (ii) Control of esotropia without glasses
        (iii) Improvement of BSV without glasses
    d. Surgery usually unnecessary

Accommodative esotropia with convergence excess   *High AC/A.*
1. Features
    a. Onset at 2–5 years
    b. Intermittent
    c. High AC/A ratio (6:1 or more)
    d. Deviation greater for near (N > D)
    e. Often hypermetropic
    f. BSV usually present
    g. Occasional microtropia
    h. Amblyopia ~~rare~~ *often !!*
2. Management
    a Full correction of hypermetropia or undercorrection of myopia
    b. Occlusion if necessary
    c. Try miotic therapy
    d. Executive bifocals in older children
    e. Orthoptic treatment
    f. Surgery usually necessary

NON-PARALYTIC STRABISMUS — EXOTROPIA

Classification
1. Primary exotropia
    a. Constant
        (i) Congenital (early onset) exotropia
        (ii) Decompensated divergence excess exotropia
    b. Intermittent
        (i) Divergence excess exotropia (distance exotropia)
        (ii) Near exotropia
2. Consecutive exotropia (following primary esotropia)
    a. Spontaneous
        (i) In late childhood or adulthood
        (ii) Usually following partially accommodative esotropia with marked hypermetropia
        (iii) Weak BSV
        (iv) Diplopia if sudden onset of exotropia
    b. Post-operative
        (i) Diplopia if sudden onset
        (ii) Usually poor or absent BSV

      (iii) More likely if esotropia was early onset
      (iv) Amblyopia
      (v) Marked hypermetropia
  c. Management
      (i) Reduce hypermetropic correction
      (ii) Base in prisms
      (iii) Orthoptic exercises to increase positive fusional
         amplitude
      (iv) Surgery for cosmesis
3. Secondary exotropia
  a. Features
      (i) In adults who have developed severe visual loss of one
         eye
      (ii) Occasionally in infants
  b. Management
      (i) Treat cause of visual loss, e.g. cataract extraction
      (ii) Pre-operative diplopia assessment
      (iii) Cosmetic surgery on defective eye in adults
      (iv) Defer surgery in children until stable

Congenital exotropia
1. Features
  a. Onset in first 6 months of life
  b. Uncommon
  c. Angle usually large and constant
  d. Often emmetropic
  e. Can have homonymous fixation
  f. Associated with mental retardation
  g. Nystagmus and DVD occur
2. Management
  a. Wait until stable
  b. Surgery usually needed

Intermittent divergence excess exotropia
1. Features
  a. 'True' if greater for distance than for near (D > N)
  b. 'Simulated' if similar for distance and near (D = N)
  c. Onset at 2–5 years
  d. Precipitated by daydreaming, tiredness, illness, alcohol (in
    adults), bright lights (often closing one eye)
  e. May have suppression or ARC
  f. May decompensate
2. Management
  a. Fully correct myopia, undercorrect hypermetropia (tinted
    glasses may help)
  b. Orthoptic exercises (anti-suppression and to increase
    fusional convergence)
  c. Most require surgery

Intermittent near exotropia
1. Features
   a. Older children and adults
   b. Asthenopia for near
   c. Poor convergence
   d. Normal retinal correspondence and fusion
   e. May be myopic
2. Management
   a. Fully correct myopia, undercorrect hypermetropia
   b. Orthoptic exercises (diplopia recognition, increasing fusional convergence)
   c. Base in prisms for near
   d. Surgery if above measures fail

Microtropia
A small angle heterotropia (usually 10 dioptres or less) in which a form of BSV exists
1. Features
   a. Often anisometropic
   b. Unequal visual acuities, with amblyopia and crowding phenomenon
   c. Fixation
      (i) Central (with manifest deviation on CT)
      (ii) Eccentric or parafoveal (no movement on CT)
   d. Binocular function
   e. Stereo tests show positive response with reduced stereo acuity
   f. Diagnosed with 4 dioptre prism test
2. Management
   a. Correct refractive error
   b. Treat amblyopia
   c. Treat any associated heterophoria

HETEROPHORIA

A latent deviation which becomes apparent when the eyes are dissociated
1. Types
   a. Exophoria — most common type
      (i) Convergence insufficiency type (N > D)
      (ii) Divergence excess type (D > N)
      (iii) Non-specific type (D = N)
   b. Esophoria
      (i) Convergence excess type (N > D)
      (ii) Divergence weakness type (D > N)
      (iii) Non-specific type (D = N)
   c. Hyperphoria — latent vertical deviation

    d. Cyclophoria — wheel rotation of eye on dissociation
       (i) Incyclophoria
      (ii) Excyclophoria
2. Symptoms (often nonspecific)
    a. Headaches
    b. Fatigue
    c. Burning, itching and redness of eyes
    d. Blurred vision relieved by closing one eye
    e. Intermittent diplopia
3. Management
    a. If fusion range greater than heterophoria, control should be achieved without treatment (similarly if fast recovery on CT)
    b. Correct refractive error
    c. Esophoria
       (i) Orthoptic treatment to improve fusional divergence
      (ii) Miotics
      (iii) Bifocals in convergence excess
      (iv) Surgery if orthoptic exercises fail or deviation too large
       (v) Prisms (BO) only as last resort
    d. Exophoria
       (i) Orthoptic treatment to improve fusional convergence
      (ii) Surgery if deviation too large
      (iii) Prisms (BI) (minimum possible) as last resort
    e. Hyperphoria
       (i) Prisms in small deviations
      (ii) Surgery if too large for prisms
      (iii) If mixed phoria correct vertical element first
    f. Cyclophoria
       (i) Correct any associated vertical phoria
      (ii) Surgery if necessary

CONVERGENCE INSUFFICIENCY

1. Types
    a. Primary — inability to obtain or maintain adequate binocular convergence
    b. Secondary — to a heterophoria, e.g. convergence insufficiency exophoria
2. Features
    a. Frontal headaches and eye strain with close work
    b. Blurred vision or intermittent diplopia for near fixation
    c. Slight exophoria for near
    d. Poor convergence
    e. Uniocular accommodation better than binocular
    f. Poor positive fusional amplitude
3. Management
    a. Correct refractive error
    b. Teach diplopia recognition

   c. Exercises to improve binocular convergence
   d. Exercises to improve relative positive convergence
   e. Teach voluntary convergence

ANOMALIES OF ACCOMMODATION

1. Accommodative spasm
   a. Features
      (i) Associated with excessive close work
      (ii) Ill-fitting or incorrect glasses
      (iii) Asthenopia
      (iv) Pseudo myopia (up to 20 D)
      (v) Constricted pupils
      (vi) Esotropia for distance and occasionally for near
   b. Aetiology
      (i) Undercorrected hypermetropia
      (ii) Exotropia
      (iii) Organic causes, e.g. cholinergic drugs, morphine,
           alcohol
      (iv) Functional, especially young women
   c. Management
      (i) Cycloplegic refraction
      (ii) Treatment with atropine for 4 weeks or more
      (iii) Stop close work
      (iv) Treat any underlying cause
2. Accommodative insufficiency
   a. Features
      (i) Asthenopia
      (ii) Blurred near vision
      (iii) Exophoria
      (iv) May have reduced convergence
   b. Aetiology
      (i) Presbyopia
      (ii) Disturbance of AC/A ratio due to correction of high
           ametropia
      (iii) After infective illnesses
      (iv) Ocular trauma
      (v) Drugs such as anticholinergics and antidepressants
   c. Management
      (i) Remove precipitating factors
      (ii) Correct significant refractive error
      (iii) May require reading glasses
      (iv) Treat any exophoria and convergence deficiency
3. Accommodative fatigue
   a. Features
      (i) Accommodation initially sufficient then deteriorates
      (ii) Similar to, but less severe than accommodative
          insufficiency

   b. Aetiology
      (i) Ill health
      (ii) Overwork
      (iii) Stress
   c. Management
      (i) Correct significant refractive error
      (ii) Treat any convergence insufficiency
      (iii) Often resolves spontaneously
4. Accommodative paralysis
   a. Features
      (i) No accommodation possible
      (ii) Blurred vision
      (iii) Micropsia
      (iv) Diplopia
   b. Aetiology
      (i) Traumatic paralysis of ciliary muscle (usually with
          traumatic mydriasis)
      (ii) Closed head injuries (including whip-lash)
      (iii) Drugs, e.g. anticholinergics (especially atropine)
      (iv) 3rd nerve palsy
      (v) Midbrain disease, e.g. pinealoma
   c. Management
      (i) Treat underlying cause
      (ii) Correct refractive error
      (iii) Give middle and near vision addition
      (iv) BI prisms may be needed

'A' AND 'V' PATTERNS

Changes in the horizontal deviation of the eyes as they move from
30 degree upgaze to 30 degree downgaze
   1. Types
      a. 'A' esotropia — increase in eso on upgaze
      b. 'A' exotropia — increase in exo on downgaze
      c. 'V' esotropia — increase in eso on downgaze
      d. 'V' exotropia — increase in exo on upgaze
Change of 10 dioptres or more for 'A' pattern, 15 dioptres or more
for 'V' pattern
   2. Features
      a. 'V' patterns are more common in eso deviations
      b. 'A' patterns are more common in exo deviations
      c. May have compensatory head posture
   3. Possible aetiologies
      a. Abnormal actions of horizontal recti in up/downgaze
      b. Abnormal actions of the cyclovertical muscles, i.e. IO, SO,
         IR, SR
   4. Surgical management
      a. For cosmesis
      b. To increase field of BSV

PARALYTIC STRABISMUS

A congenital or acquired incomitant deviation of the visual axes resulting from limitation of ocular movement

Types
1. Neurogenic
2. Mechanical
3. Myogenic

Neurogenic strabismus
1. Unilateral nerve palsies
    a. 3rd cranial nerve palsies
    b. 4th cranial nerve palsies
    c. 6th cranial nerve palsies
2. Single muscle palsies
    a. Medial rectus
        (i) Rare
        (ii) Differentiate from atypical Duane's
        (iii) Exotropia (N > D)
        (iv) Face turn to opposite side
    b. Inferior rectus
        (i) Rare
        (ii) Differentiate from mechanical restriction
        (iii) Hypertropia and slight exotropia
        (iv) Head tilt to opposite side, face turn to affected side, chin down
    c. Superior rectus
        (i) Rare
        (ii) Underaction common in a V-esotropia
        (iii) Hypotropia (D > N) and slight exotropia
        (iv) Chin up with head tilt and face turn to affected side
    d. Inferior oblique
        (i) Very rare
        (ii) Differentiate, from Brown's syndrome
3. Bilateral nerve palsies
    a. Bilateral 6th nerve palsy
        (i) Large alternating esotropia (D > N) with 6th crossed fixation
        (ii) No BSV possible
        (iii) Sequelae. Bilateral contracture of MR
    b. Bilateral 4th nerve palsy
        (i) V-esotropia if acquired
        (ii) Extorsion and hypertropia (N > D)
        (iii) Usually asymmetrical with hypertropia in primary position on more affected side
        (iv) Hypertropia may reverse between laevodepression and dextrodepression
        (v) Chin down if symmetrical
        (vi) Head tilt to side of more affected eye if asymmetrical

　　　　(vii) Small field of BSV (if any)
　　　　(viii) Sequelae. Bilateral overaction of IR

Management of neurogenic strabismus
　1. Congenital palsies
　　　a. Surgery if large CHP or manifest strabismus
　　　b. Delay surgery until 4–5 years old
　　　c. In adults, no treatment if symptomless
　2. Acquired palsies
　　　a. Exclude treatable cause
　　　b. Wait until stable (6 months)
　　　c. Prisms if small deviation or medically unfit
　　　d. Botulinum toxin to antagonist to prevent contracture and
　　　　fibrosis
　3. Surgical principles
　　　a. Aim to relieve symptoms
　　　b. Increase field of BSV (mostly in primary position and in
　　　　down gaze)
　　　c. Weaken the ipsilateral antagonist
　　　d. Strengthen the palsied muscle (if some action remains)
　　　e. Weaken the overacting yoke muscle

Mechanical strabismus
　1. Features
　　　a. Ductions and versions are equally limited (in neurogenic
　　　　palsies versions are usually less limited than ductions)
　　　b. Movement often limited in opposite directions of gaze
　　　c. Muscle sequelae are confined to overaction of contralateral
　　　　eye in the direction of the limitation of movement
　　　d. Abnormal movement patterns may result
　　　e. Saccadic velocity is normal until the point of mechanical
　　　　restriction is reached
　　　f. Forced duction test shows restricted passive movements
　　　g. Globe retraction and rise in intraocular pressure can occur
　　　　on attempted movement against the restriction
　2. Types
　　　a. Congenital
　　　　　(i)   Strabismus fixus. Fibrosis and contracture of both MR.
　　　　　　　Marked esotropia
　　　　　(ii) Generalised fibrosis syndrome. Ptosis and marked
　　　　　　　bilateral downwards deviation
　　　　　(iii) Congenital adherence syndromes, e.g. abnormal fascial
　　　　　　　connections
　　　　　(iv) Brown's syndrome
　　　b. Acquired
　　　　　(i)   Dysthyroid eye disease. Myopathic and later mechanical
　　　　　　　restriction (usually IR, MR and SR)
　　　　　(ii) Orbital injuries, e.g. blow out fractures

3. Management
   a. No treatment if asymptomatic or cosmetically acceptable
   b. Prisms
   c. Botulinum toxin to contralateral synergist
   d. Surgery
      (i) To produce or enlarge field of BSV in straight ahead and down gaze positions
      (ii) To improve cosmesis
      (iii) To reduce any anomalous ocular movements
      (iv) To improve compensatory head posture
      (v) Recess tight muscles
      (vi) Weaken overacting contralateral synergists

Myogenic strabismus
1. Types
   a. Myasthenia gravis
   b. Dysthyroid myopathy
   c. Ocular myopathies
   d. Ocular myositis
2. Management
   a. Treat underlying disease
   b. Surgery usually contraindicated both for ophthalmoplegia and ptosis (risk of corneal exposure)
   c. Relieving prisms
   d. Occlusion to overcome diplopia
   e. Ptosis props

SPECIAL OCULAR MOTILITY SYNDROMES
Brown's syndrome (superior oblique tendon sheath syndrome)
1. Features
   a. Congenital or acquired in early childhood
   b. Limitation of active and passive elevation in adduction
   c. Down drift of affected eye in adduction (palpebral fissure may widen)
   d. 'V' pattern common
   e. Unilateral or bilateral
   f. If unilateral, CHP of chin elevation and head tilt to affected side
   g. Diagnosed with forced duction test
   h. May 'click'
   i. Often spontaneously improves in late childhood or early teens
   j. Occasionally acquired in adulthood
2. Aetiology
   a. Congenital
      (i) Tight SO anterior tendon sheath

      (ii) Short SO muscle and tendon
      (iii) Nodule on SO tendon
      (iv) Anomalous innervation
  b. Acquired
      (i) Inflammation
      (ii) Trauma
      (iii) SO plication
3. Management
  a. If congenital, most have compensated or improve spontaneously
  b. If marked CHP or decompensation, consider surgery
  c. If acquired, local steroids or prisms may help

Duane's retraction syndrome

1. Classification
  Type A
  a. Reduced or absent abduction of one eye with face turn to that side
  b. Widening of palpebral fissure on abduction
  c. Narrowing of palpebral fissure and retraction of globe on adduction
  d. Less marked limitation of adduction
  e. Poor convergence
  Type B
    Limited abduction but normal adduction
  Type C
  a. Adduction more limited than abduction
  b. Face turn to the opposite side
  c. Exotropia

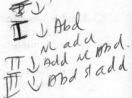

A or V patterns seen, unilateral or bilateral
Can have associated skeletal, facial and neural abnormalities
2. Ocular associations
  a. Colobomata
  b. Heterochromia iridis
  c. Lens opacities
  d. Microphthalmos
  e. Persistent pupillary membrane
3. Possible aetiologies
  a. Congenital
      (i) Aplasia or dysplasia of VI nerve nucleus
      (ii) More generalized brainstem dysplasia
      (iii) Mechanical abnormalities of horizontal recti
  b. Acquired
      (i) Excessive lateral rectus resection
      (ii) Localized inflammation
      (iii) Orbital trauma
4. Management
  a. Conservative (the majority)

    b. Surgical only if
        (i) Large CHP
        (ii) Decompensation
        (iii) Large strabismus

Mobius' syndrome
1. Features
    a. Rare, congenital *(8th)*
    b. Aplasia of the 6th, 7th, 9th and 12th cranial nerve nuclei
    c. Horizontal gaze palsies
    d. Lower facial muscles often spared
    e. High refractive errors are common
    f. Mental retardation
    g. Deafness
    h. Pectoral muscle hypoplasia
    i. Limb malformations
2. Management
    a. Correct significant refractive errors
    b. Treat amblyopia
    c. Avoid surgery unless cosmetically unacceptable strabismus

Double elevator palsy
1. Features
    a. Unilateral, congenital   *Extra lid fold LL.*
    b. Due to ipsilateral paresis of SR and IO
    c. Restriction of elevation in abduction and adduction
    d. Hypotropia with pseudoptosis
    e. Chin up CHP
2. Management   *R/O restrictive IR*
    a. Conservative   *Do FDT*
    b. Surgical only if
        (i) Gross CHP
        (ii) Large strabismus

Neuro-ophthalmology

OPTIC NERVE

1. Features
   a. 45 mm long
      (i) 1 mm intraocular
      (ii) 30 mm intraorbital
      (iii) 6 mm in optic canal
      (iv) 10 mm intracranial
   b. Contains one million myelinated fibres
   c. Only myelinated up to lamina cribosa
   d. Disc composed of 50% glial tissue, 50% ganglion cell axons
2. Relations
   a. Embraced by muscle cone
   b. Ciliary ganglion lies laterally
   c. Orbital portion crossed over by
      (i) Nasociliary nerve
      (ii) Ophthalmic artery
3. Blood supply
   a. Pial vessels
      (i) Ophthalmic artery
      (ii) Internal carotid artery
      (iii) Anterior cerebral artery
   b. Branches of central retinal artery
   c. Posterior ciliary arteries

OPTIC CHIASM

1. Features
   a. Decussation of nasal fibres
   b. Lower nasal fibres loop forward into opposite optic nerve
      (anterior knee of Willibrand)
2. Relations
   a. Chiasm lies above sella in 80% (fixed), anteriorly in 10%
      (prefixed), posteriorly in 10% (postfixed)
   b. Inferior — diaphragma sellae
   c. Superior — lamina terminalis

197

    d. Anterior — anterior cerebral and communicating arteries
    e. Posterior — pituitary stalk
    f. Lateral — internal carotid artery
3. Blood supply
    a. Internal carotid artery
    b. Anterior cerebral artery

OPTIC TRACT

1. Features
    a. Continuation of optic pathway
    b. Projects to
        (i) Lateral geniculate body (visual fibres)
        (ii) Both pretectal nuclei (light reflex fibres)
        (iii) Superior colliculus (ocular reflex movements)
2. Relations
    a. Anterolateral — anterior perforated substance
    b. Posteriomedial — pituitary stalk
    c. Inferior — posterior cerebral artery
3. Blood supply
    a. Anterior choroidal artery
    b. Posterior communicating artery

LATERAL GENICULATE BODY

1. Features
    a. Receives optic tract
    b. Contains synapses
    c. Saddle-shaped
    d. 6 layers centred on hilum
    e. Crossed fibres project to layers 1, 4, 6
    f. Uncrossed to layers 2, 3, 5
    g. Projects to visual cortex
2. Blood supply
    a. Posterior communicating artery
    b. Anterior choroidal artery

OPTIC RADIATION

1. Features
    a. Myelinated nerve fibres
    b. Connect lateral geniculate body and occipital cortex
    c. Passes in posterior limb of internal capsule
    d. Passes forwards and laterally anterior to lateral ventricle
    e. Lower fibres sweep forward into temporal lobe (Meyer's loop)
2. Blood supply
    a. Anterior choroidal artery

b. Deep optic branches of middle cerebral artery
c. Perforating vessels of calcarine artery (branch of posterior cerebral artery)

VISUAL CORTEX

1. Features
   a. Medial aspect of occipital lobe
   b. Above and below calcarine fissure
   c. Extends laterally to lunate sulcus
   d. Characterized by stria of Gennari
   e. Macula represented posteriorly
   f. Upper gyrus represents lower field
   g. 6 layers
      (i) Laminar zonalis
      (ii) Outer granular
      (iii) Laminar pyrimidalis
      (iv) Inner granular
      (v) Ganglion layer
      (vi) Laminar multiformis
2. Blood supply
   a. Calcarine branch of posterior cerebral artery
   b. Some middle cerebral supply to occipital pole

OCULOMOTOR NERVE (3rd)

1. Features
   a. Motor to superior, inferior and medial recti
   b. Motor to inferior oblique and levator palpebrae superioris
   c. Parasympathetic supply to ciliary body and sphincter pupillae
2. Nuclei
   a. Paired subnuclei to individual muscles
   b. At level of superior colliculus
   c. Unpaired caudal subnucleus to levator palpebrae superioris
   d. Pupillomotor nucleus (Edinger–Westphal)
   e. Superior rectus subnucleus supplies contralateral muscle
3. Fasciculus
   a. Passes ventrally through red nucleus
   b. Emerges into interpeduncular fossa
   c. Between superior cerebellar and posterior cerebral arteries
4. Nerve
   a. Passes forward below optic tract
   b. Lateral to posterior communicating artery
   c. Enters lateral wall of cavernous sinus
   d. Receives sympathetic supply from internal carotid plexus
   e. Divides into upper and lower divisions

   f. Passes through superior orbital fissure (within tendinous ring)
   g. Upper division supplies
      (i) Superior rectus
     (ii) Levator palpebrae superioris
   h. Lower division supplies
      (i) Inferior and medial rectus
     (ii) Inferior oblique (with parasympathetic branch to ciliary ganglion)

TROCHLEAR NERVE (4th)

1. Features
   a. Pure motor nerve
   b. Supplies superior oblique
   c. Longest cranial nerve (7.5 cm)
   d. Only cranial nerve to emerge dorsally
2. Nucleus
   a. In dorsal midbrain
   b. At level of inferior colliculus
3. Fasciculus
   a. Passes dorsally
   b. Decussates
   c. Emerges below inferior colliculus
4. Nerve
   a. Passes round midbrain
   b. Between posterior cerebral and superior cerebellar arteries
   c. Passes beneath free edge of tentorium
   d. Enters lateral wall of cavernous sinus
   e. Enters orbit via superior orbital fissure (outside tendinous ring)
   f. Passes medially along orbital roof to superior oblique

TRIGEMINAL NERVE (5th)

1. Features
   a. Sensory to face and eye
   b. Motor to muscles of mastication
2. Nuclei
   a. Mesencephalic (midbrain). Proprioception
   b. Sensory (pontine). Light touch, pressure
   c. Spinal (medulla to cervical spine). Pain, temperature
   d. Motor (pontine)
3. Nerve
   a. Emerges from ventral pons
   b. Large sensory root
   c. Small motor root
   d. Passes below tentorium to ganglion

4. Ganglion
   a. Cell bodies of sensory cells (except proprioception)
   b. Extradural in Meckel's cave
   c. Receives
      (i) Ophthalmic division
      (ii) Maxillary division
      (iii) Mandibular division
5. Ophthalmic division (5a)
   a. In lateral wall of cavernous sinus
   b. Divides into
      (i) Lacrimal nerve
      (ii) Frontal nerve
      (iii) Nasociliary nerve
   c. Supplies sensation to upper face including eye
   d. 5 branches of nasociliary nerve
      (i) Sensory root of ciliary ganglion
      (ii) 2–3 long ciliary nerves
      (iii) Posterior ethmoidal nerve
      (iv) Anterior ethmoidal nerve
      (v) Infratrochlear nerve
6. Maxillary division (5b)
   a. Lies in lateral wall of cavernous sinus
   b. Exits cranium via foramen rotundum
   c. Sensory supply to middle of face including inferior
      conjunctiva
7. Mandibular division (5c)
   a. Leaves cranium via foramen ovale
   b. Sensory to inferior face
   c. Motor to muscles of mastication

ABDUCENT NERVE (6th)

1. Features
   Motor to lateral rectus
2. Nucleus
   a. Near midline in lower pons
   b. Beneath facial colliculus
3. Fasciculus
   a. Passes ventrally
   b. Exits in pontomedullary groove
4. Nerve
   a. Passes upward through cisterna pontis
   b. Pierces dura
   c. Passes over apex of petrous bone
   d. Enters cavernous sinus
   e. Enters orbit through superior orbital fissure
   f. Lies within the tendinous ring
   g. Passes laterally to supply lateral rectus

FACIAL NERVE (7th)

1. Features
   a. Motor to
      (i) Muscles of facial expression
      (ii) Stylohyoid
      (iii) Posterior belly of digastric
      (iv) Stapedius
   b. Secretomotor to lacrimal and salivary glands
   c. Taste to anterior two thirds of tongue
2. Nucleus
   a. In lower pons
   b. Beneath floor of fourth ventricle
3. Fasciculus
   a. Passes round abducent nucleus
   b. Exits ventrally from pontomedullary junction
4. Nerve
   a. Enters internal auditory canal
   b. Geniculate ganglion contains cell bodies of chorda tympani (taste)
   c. Branches within cranium
      (i) Chorda tympani
      (ii) Greater superficial petrosal nerve
      (iii) Nerve to stapedius
      (iv) Branches to tympanic plexus
   d. Exits from stylomastoid foramen
   e. Initial branches
      (i) Posterior auricular nerve
      (ii) Tympanic nerve
   f. Branches in parotid gland
      (i) Temporal
      (ii) Zygomatic
      (iii) Buccal
      (iv) Mandibular
      (v) Cervical

Ciliary ganglion

1. Features
   a. Small parasympathetic ganglion (3 mm long)
   b. Lies 1 cm from optic foramen
   c. Between optic nerve and lateral rectus
   d. Contains parasympathetic synapse
2. Receives
   a. Long sensory root from nasociliary nerve
   b. Short parasympathetic root (motor to ciliary body and sphincter pupillae)
   c. Slender sympathetic root (supply to vasculature and dilator pupillae)
3. Branches — 6–7 short ciliary nerves to globe

Pupilloconstrictor pathway
1. Afferents pass in optic nerve and tract
2. Synapse in the pretectal nucleus
3. Project to both Edinger-Westphal nuclei
4. Efferents pass in the 3rd nerve
5. Lie dorsally and laterally in nerve
6. Pass with branch to inferior oblique
7. Synapse in ciliary ganglion
8. Postganglionic fibres pass in short ciliary nerves to sphincter pupillae

Pupilloconstrictor pathway
1. Sympathetic nervous system
2. Originates in posterior hypothalamus
3. Descends to T_1 level
4. Synapses in lateral horn
5. Efferent exits with the ventral root
6. Leaves the spinal nerve in the white ramus
7. Enters the sympathetic chain
8. Ascends and synapses in the superior cervical ganglion
9. Postganglionic fibres pass in carotid plexus
10. Transfer to 5a in cavernous sinus
11. Pass via long ciliary nerves to pupillodilator muscle

Horizontal gaze centre
1. Situated in paramedian pontine reticular formation (PPRF)
2. At level of 6th nerve nucleus
3. Controls horizontal gaze to ipsilateral side
4. Projects to
   a. Ipsilateral 6th nerve nucleus
   b. 3rd nerve nucleus (via contralateral medial longitudinal fasciculus)

Vertical gaze centre
1. Poorly understood
2. Pretectal and rostral mesencephalic reticular formation
3. Acts bilaterally

Vergence centre
1. 3 defined areas
2. Similar to vertical gaze centre
3. Defects associated clinically with vertical gaze palsies

Medial longitudinal fasciculus (MLF)
1. Near midline
2. Extending from anterior horn cells of spinal cord to thalamus
3. Connects
   a. Oculomotor nuclei
   b. Gaze centres

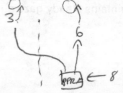

OCULAR MOVEMENTS

1. Saccade
   a. Refixation movement
   b. Latency 200 ms
   c. Velocity 200–700°/s (fast)
   d. Controlled by
      (i) Frontal cortex — *contralateral!* [Sacc]: [Pers.] Front: Occip
      (ii) Superior colliculus
   e. Defects
      (i) Delayed
      (ii) Slow
      (iii) Hypermetric (overshoot)
      (iv) Hypometric (undershoot)
   f. Tests
      (i) Refixation
      (ii) Rotation
      (iii) Calorics
      (iv) Optokinetic nystagmus (fast saccadic return phase)
2. Pursuits
   a. Conjugate movement
   b. Maintaining foveal fixation
   c. Latency 125 ms
   d. Velocity less than 50°/s (relatively slow) *slow .*
   e. Controlled by occipital lobe *ipsilatere .*
   f. Defect — reduced (saccadic pursuit)
   g. Tests
      (i) Dolls head
      (ii) Rotation
      (iii) Optokinetic nystagmus (smooth pursuit phase)
3. Vergence
   a. Disjunctive movement
   b. Maintaining foveal fixation on object approach
   c. Latency 160 ms
   d. Velocity less than 20°/s (slow)
   e. Controlled by
      (i) Frontal and occipital lobes
      (ii) Possibly midbrain centre
   f. Types
      (i) Voluntary
      (ii) Accommodative
      (iii) Proximal induced
      (iv) Tonic
      (v) Fusional
   g. Test — look from distance to near
4. Vestibulo-ocular movements
   a. Smooth conjugate movement
   b. Maintains steady gaze during head movement

c. Latency 100 ms
d. Peak velocity 300–400°/s
e. Utricle and saccule respond to rectilinear acceleration
f. Semicircular canals respond to rotational acceleration
g. Mediated by vestibular nuclei projecting to PPRF
h. Also input from neck proprioceptors
i. Defects cause oscillopsia
j. Tests
   (i) Calorics
   (ii) Rotation

EMBRYOLOGY OF THE VISUAL PATHWAY

1. Primitive optic vesicle (neuroectodermal)
2. Forms as diverticulum from diencephalon
3. Proximal part forms optic stalk
4. Distal part invaginates to form optic vesicle
5. Optic vesicle forms retina
6. Ganglion cell axons converge and invade optic stalk
7. Medullation of axons proceeds in retrograde direction
8. Mesoderm forms dura, arachnoid and pia

THE PUPILS

Pupil examination
1. Size, symmetry, shape
2. Reactions (brisk, sluggish)
3. Direct reaction
4. Consensual reaction
5. Near reaction
6. Relative afferent pupillary defect
7. Associated ocular examination, e.g. ocular movements, upper lid position, ophthalmoscopy
8. Pharmacological tests

Pupil abnormalities
1. Essential anisocoria
   a. Up to 20% prevalence in normal population
   b. Unknown cause
   c. Normal pupil reflexes
2. Persistent pupillary fibres
   a. Congenital
   b. Remnants of pupillary membrane
3. Iris Coloboma
   a. Congenital
   b. Total or partial
   c. Pigment frill present

4. Corectopia
   a. Congenital displacement of pupil
   b. Associated with peripheral anterior synechiae
5. Polycoria
   a. Multiple true pupils
   b. Rare
6. Acquired pupil irregularity
   a. Posterior synechiae
   b. Traumatic mydriasis
   c. Iris melanoma
   d. Sphincter infarction
   e. Iridectomy
   f. Iris prolapse
   g. Iridodialysis
7. Horner's syndrome
   a. Features
      (i) Ptosis (2 mm only)
      (ii) Miosis
      (iii) Preganglionic type associated with anhydrosis of upper
            face
      (iv) Iris heterochromia (if congenital or longstanding)
   b. Causes
      (i) Congenital
      (ii) Interruption of sympathetic pathway (via T_1)
      (iii) Thalamic, internal capsule or brainstem lesions, e.g.
            disseminated sclerosis, glioma, vascular lesions
      (iv) Cervical cord lesions, e.g. syringomyelia, glioma,
            ependymoma
      (v) T_1 root lesions, e.g. Pancoast tumour, cervical rib,
          avulsion injury
      (vi) Cervical sympathetic chain lesions, e.g. Hodgkin's
           disease, carotid aneurysm, carotid body tumour
      (vii) Internal carotid artery or cavernous sinus lesions
   c. Tests
      (i) 1% Hydroxyamphetamine drops dilate pupil only in
          preganglionic lesion
      (ii) 1% Phenylephrine drops dilate pupil in postganglionic
           lesions
8. Tonic pupil (Adie's)   *Light/Near dis - very slow though.*
   a. Young adults
   b. Dilated pupil
   c. Tonic reaction to light and accommodation
   d. Sectorial vermiform movements
   e. Constricts with 0.125% pilocarpine or 2.5% methacholine
   f. Possibly post viral degeneration of ciliary ganglion
   g. Associated with hyporeflexia (Holmes–Adie syndrome)
9. Argyll–Robertson pupil
   a. Bilaterally small irregular pupils

— b. Light near dissociation
   c. Causes
      (i) Syphilis
      (ii) Diabetes mellitus *
      (iii) Encephalitis
10. Parinaud's syndrome
   a. Bilateral mid-dilated pupils
— b. Light/near dissociation
   c. Convergence retraction nystagmus
   d. Poor upgaze
   e. Staring facies (Collier's sign)
   f. Causes
      (i) Pinealoma   1 y/o.
      (ii) Teratoma of pineal gland   10 y/o.   trauma 20 y/o
      (iii) Multiple sclerosis   30 y/o.
      (iv) Vascular lesions   40 y/o.   – stroke 50 y/o.
11. 3rd nerve palsy (complete)
   a. Dilated fixed pupil
   b. Abducted and slightly depressed eye
   c. Ptosis
12. Marcus Gunn Pupil
   a. Normal sized pupils
   b. Relative afferent pupillary defect (RAPD) on swinging light test
   c. Caused by optic nerve or severe retinal disease
13. Drug-induced pupil abnormality
   a. Common cause
   b. Topical
      (i) Cycloplegics
      (ii) Mydriatics
      (iii) Miotics
   c. Systemic
      (i) Constricted by opiates
      (ii) Dilated by anticholinergics, antidepressants, amphetamines
14. Disorders of Light/near dissociation
   a. Features
      (i) Absent or reduced light reaction
      (ii) Near reaction present
   b. Causes
      (i) Parinaud's syndrome
      (ii) Argyll–Robertson
      (iii) Holmes–Adie   – slow!
      (iv) Aberrant 3rd nerve regeneration
      (v) Diabetes mellitus   young-
      (vi) Dystrophia myotonica

OPTIC DISC ABNORMALITIES

1. Congenital optic pit
   a. Often inferotemporal and unilateral
   b. Associated with serous macular detachment
   c. Arcuate scotomata and other field defects occur
2. Optic disc coloboma
   a. Deep excavation
   b. May produce various field defects
   c. Vision normal or reduced
3. 'Morning glory' syndrome
   a. Unilateral dysplastic coloboma
   b. Cup filled with glial tissue
   c. Cup surrounded by pigment ring
   d. Spoke-like radiation of vessels
   e. Poor vision
   f. Retinal detachment occurs
4. Tilted disc
   a. Often bilateral
   b. Associated with
      (i) High myopia
      (ii) Astigmatism
      (iii) Field defects
5. Optic nerve hypoplasia
   a. Small disc with pale halo
   b. Poor vision
   c. Various field defects
   d. RAPD if unilateral
   e. Associated with
      (i) Aniridia
      (ii) De Morsier's syndrome
      (iii) Microphthalmos
6. Myelinated nerve fibres
   a. Congenital
   b. White flame shaped patches
   c. Usually adjacent to disc
   d. Enlarged blind spot
7. Melanocytoma
   a. Benign melanotic disc lesion
   b. Often inferiorly
   c. Usually in dark-skinned races
   d. Normal vision
8. Optic disc drusen
   a. Congenital, often familial
   b. 70% bilateral
   c. Absent optic cup
   d. Multiple opalescent bodies
   e. Autofluorescence

    f. Increasing prominence with age
    g. Associated with
       (i) Vitreous haemorrhage
      (ii) SRNVM
     (iii) Angioid streaks
     (iv) Retinitis pigmentosa
9. Bergmeister's papilla
    a. Remnant of glial sheath of hyaloid artery
    b. Vision unaffected

CAUSES OF OPTIC DISC SWELLING

1. Papilloedema – *Bilateral*
2. Papillitis –
3. Malignant hypertension
4. Focal choroiditis
5. Central retinal vein occlusion
6. Ischaemic optic neuropathy
7. Optic nerve compression – *on meningioma, glioma*
8. Infiltrative optic neuropathy, e.g. lymphoma – *± bilateral.*
9. Ocular hypotony
10. Toxic optic neuropathy – *bilateral.*
11. Optic disc drusen and hypermetropia (pseudoswelling) //
    – *uveitis, papillophlebitis, Lyme disease!!*

Papilloedema
1. Features
    a. Disc swelling in the presence of raised intracranial pressure
    b. Vision usually good until late stages
    c. Obscurations may occur
2. Stages
    a. Early
       (i) Absent spontaneous venous pulsation
      (ii) Nerve fibre swelling at disc
     (iii) Disc capillary plexus dilatation
     (iv) Peripapillary haemorrhage
      (v) Retinal folds
    b. Acute decompensated
       (i) Grossly swollen hyperaemic disc
      (ii) Masking of blood vessels
     (iii) Loss of cup
     (iv) Haemorrhages
      (v) Cotton wool spots
    c. Chronic
       (i) Champagne cork appearance
      (ii) Fewer haemorrhages
     (iii) Macular star
     (iv) Arcuate field loss (late)

   d. Terminal
      (i) Pale atrophied flat disc
      (ii) Arteriolar attenuation
      (iii) Poor vision

Optic neuritis
1. Features
   a. Inflammatory lesion
   b. Reduced vision
   c. Paracentral or central scotoma
   d. Pain with ocular movement
   e. Colour desaturation
   f. Uhthoff's phenomenon
   g. Pulfrich's phenomenon
   h. Relative afferent pupillary defect
   i. Increased latency on VER
2. Types
   a. Papillitis
      (i) Disc swelling
      (ii) Hyperaemia
      (iii) Haemorrhages
   b. Retrobulbar neuritis. Normal disc
   c. Neuroretinitis
      (i) Papillitis
      (ii) Macular star —(Lebers particularly) stellate Neuroretin
                                          NOT assoc c̄ MS!
3. Causes
   a. Multiple sclerosis (commonest cause)
   b. Viral diseases of childhood, e.g. Devic's disease
   c. Viral encephalitis
   d. Infectious mononucleosis
   e. Herpes zoster ophthalmicus
   f. Contiguous inflammation of orbit, meninges or sinuses
   g. Granulomatous inflammation of optic nerve, e.g. syphilis,
      TB, sarcoid
   h. Intraocular inflammation

Optic atrophy
1. Congenital or hereditary (primary)
   a. Leber's optic atrophy —(3♀?)
   b. Dominant and recessive types
   c. Infantile optic atrophy
   d. Congenital syphilis
2. Secondary to raised intracranial pressure
3. Secondary to retinal disease (consecutive)
   a. Vascular, e.g. central retinal artery occlusion
   b. Inflammatory, e.g. Behçet's
   c. Choroiditis
   d. Retinitis pigmentosa

4. Secondary to optic neuritis or neuropathy
   a. Vascular, e.g. ischaemic optic neuropathy
   b. Multiple sclerosis
   c. Vitamin B_1 deficiency
   d. Toxic neuropathy, e.g. drugs, heavy metals   _lead, ethambutol, INH_
   e. Infection, e.g. syphilis   _methanol, Entrovuform,_
   f. Glaucoma   _Lebers Op. Neuropen._   _tobacco /alohol (36,12)_
5. Secondary to optic nerve compression
   a. Tumours, e.g. meningioma, pituitary adenoma
   b. Aneurysm
   c. Dysthyroid eye disease
   d. Infiltrative disease, e.g. sarcoid, lymphoma
   e. Infection, e.g. orbital cellulitis
   f. Bony overgrowth, e.g. Paget's disease
6. Secondary to trauma
7. Secondary to metabolic disease, e.g. mucopolysaccharidoses

CHIASMAL LESIONS

1. Pituitary tumours
   a. Middle-aged adults. Males = Females
   b. Present with visual failure and/or hormonal imbalance
   c. Chromophobe commonest (often prolactinoma)
   d. Chromophobe or basophil can secrete ACTH (Cushing's disease)
   e. Eosinophil can secrete GH (gigantism or acromegaly)
   f. 30% tumours nonfunctioning
   g. Bitemporal hemianopia and optic atrophy
   h. Large pituitary fossa, double floor sign, bony erosion on SXR
   i. Treatment
      (i) Dopamine antagonists for prolactinoma and to a lesser extent acromegaly
      (ii) Correct hormone deficiencies
      (iii) Surgery (usually transphenoidal)
      (iv) Radiotherapy (larger adenomas)
2. Meningioma
   a. Adults (especially middle-aged women)
   b. Present with visual failure
   c. Situated at sphenoidal ridge, tuberculum sella, olfactory groove
   d. Often asymmetrical field loss, e.g. junctional scotoma
   e. Optic atrophy
   f. Hyperostosis seen on SXR
   g. Surgical treatment
   h. Good prognosis if excision complete

3. Craniopharyngioma
   a. Children and young adults. Males = Females
   b. Present with features of raised intracranial pressure, hormonal imbalance or visual failure
   c. Various patterns of field loss
   d. Papilloedema or optic atrophy
   e. Slow growing, often cystic
   f. Calcification shows on SXR
   g. Surgical treatment
   h. Less good prognosis
4. Aneurysms
   a. Middle-aged adults. Males = Females
   b. Present with visual failure and/or ophthalmoplegia
   c. Internal carotid, anterior communicating or ophthalmic arteries
   d. Field loss depends on position of lesion
   e. Calcification or bony erosion on SXR
   f. Surgical treatment
   g. Variable prognosis
5. Optic nerve or chiasmal glioma
   a. Children (80% are under 10)
   b. 60% have von Recklinghausen's disease
   c. Present with visual loss
   d. Field loss depends on position of lesion
   e. Optic atrophy (occasional papilloedema)
   f. Very slow growing
   g. Enlarged optic foramen on SXR
   h. Observe (occasional radiotherapy or surgery)
6. Other chiasmal lesions
   a. Multiple sclerosis
   b. Trauma
   c. Basal meningitis or arachnoiditis
   d. Sphenoidal sinus mucocoele or carcinoma
   e. Pituitary infarction (apoplexy)
   f. Empty-sella syndrome

RETROCHIASMAL LESIONS

All have homonymous field defects
A total homonymous hemianopia has no localizing value
Lesions of optic tract and lateral geniculate body produce incongruous field loss
Visual acuity usually unaffected
1. Optic tract lesions
   a. Features
      (i) Rare
      (ii) Incongruous hemianopic field loss

b. Causes
   (i) Posteriorly extending chiasmal lesions
   (ii) Vascular lesions
2. Temporal lobe lesions
   a. Features
      (i) Affecting Meyer's loop
      (ii) Causing upper homonymous quadrantanopia
      (iii) If incongruous, denser on nasal side
   b. Causes
      (i) Gliomas
      (ii) Vascular lesions
      (iii) Surgical trauma
3. Parietal lobe lesions
   a. Features
      (i) Complete homonymous hemianopia
      (ii) Occasionally lower quadrantanopia
      (iii) Decreased optokinetic nystagmus on side of lesion
      (iv) Associated with apraxia
   b. Causes
      (i) Metastases
      (ii) Glioma
      (iii) Meningioma
      (iv) Middle cerebral artery thrombosis
4. Occipital lobe lesions
   a. Features
      (i) Congruous homonymous hemianopia
      (ii) May have macular sparing
   b. Causes
      (i) Vascular (90%)
      (ii) Tumours
      (iii) Post traumatic (contrecoup)

NUCLEAR AND INFRANUCLEAR PALSIES

Oculomotor (3rd) nerve palsies
1. Features
   a. May be complete, pupil sparing or combined with sympathetic paralysis
   b. Ptosis
   c. Fixed dilated pupil (if complete)
   d. Eye abducted and depressed
2. Nuclear lesions
   a. Vascular, demyelination
   b. Usually incomplete
   c. Unilateral 3rd nerve palsy with contralateral superior rectus palsy
   d. Bilateral with sparing of levator palpebrae superioris

3. Fascicular lesions
   a. Vascular, demyelination or tumour
   b. Weber's syndrome (3rd nerve palsy and contralateral hemiparesis)
   c. Benedikt's syndrome (3rd nerve palsy and contralateral cerebellar signs)
4. Interpeduncular lesions
   a. Posterior communicating artery aneurysm — *pupil involvd.*
   b. Usually painful and complete
   c. Other causes — trauma, meningitis, raised intracranial pressure
5. Cavernous sinus lesions
   a. Aneurysm, thrombosis, fistula, extrasellar pituitary tumour
   b. Often combined with 4th, 5th, 6th nerve palsies
   c. May be paralysis of pupillary sympathetics
6. Superior orbital fissure, orbital apex and orbital lesions
   a. Tumours, granulomatous infiltrate, trauma, orbital cellulitis, dysthyroid eye disease
   b. Proptosis
   c. May be combined with 4th, 5th, 6th nerve palsies
7. Other causes of 3rd nerve palsy
   a. Diabetes mellitus (often pupil sparing)
   b. Arteriosclerosis
   c. Autoimmune vasculitis   *myaesVaenia gr.*
   d. Herpes zoster ophthalmicus
   e. Migraine
8. Aberrant 3rd nerve regeneration
   a. Several patterns
   b. Lid elevation on downgaze or adduction
   c. Adduction or retraction on down or upgaze
   d. Various ocular movements producing miosis

Trochlear (4th) nerve palsies
1. Features
   a. Oblique diplopia, worse on downgaze
   b. Hypertropia (greater for near)
   c. Head tilt and face turn to opposite side with chin down
   d. Commonest causes are trauma and vascular (hypertension, diabetes)
2. Bielschowsky test — hypertropia on tilting head to side of lesion
3. Types
   a. Isolated — unilateral or bilateral (usually traumatic)
   b. Associated with other palsies
   c. Complicated (dorsal midbrain lesions)

Abducent (6th) nerve palsies
1. Features
   a. Horizontal diplopia (greater for distance)
   b. Complete or partial failure of abduction
   c. Face turn towards affected side
   d. Esotropia
2. Types
   a. Isolated
   b. Associated with other palsies
   c. Complicated (pontine lesions)

Aetiology of ocular nerve palsies
1. Idiopathic (25%) ~50% recover
2. Infarction. (3rd, 4th) Diabetes mellitus, hypertension 6^R also.
3. Trauma (4th) ~ also 3, 6th
4. Pressure from aneurysm (3rd) — rarely others?
5. Multiple sclerosis (6th, 3rd)
6. Pressure from neoplasia → meningioma / Nasoph. Ca, post glioma
7. Tentorial herniation (3rd)
8. Inflammations
   a. Basal meningitis
   b. Herpes zoster ophthalmicus
   c. Vasculitis
   d. Sarcoidosis
   e. Acute infections
   f. Polyneuropathy
9. Raised intracranial pressure (3rd, 4th) RTC →6^R bilat.
10. Caroticocavernous fistulae (multiple palsies)
11. Ophthalmoplegic migraine
12. Congenital

HORIZONTAL GAZE PALSIES

1. Congenital oculomotor apraxia
   a. Bilateral saccadic paralysis
   b. Associated with head thrusting
2. Mobius syndrome
   a. Horizontal gaze palsy
   b. 6th, 7th, 8th, 9th nerve palsies
3. Focal frontal lesions
   Contralateral saccadic palsy
4. Focal parieto-occipital lesions
   Ipsilateral pursuit palsy ('cog-wheel' pursuit)
5. Focal tegmental lesion
   Ipsilateral pursuit and saccadic palsy
6. Focal pontine lesion (PPRF)
   Ipsilateral horizontal gaze palsy

7. Diffuse lesions
    a. Parkinson's disease
    b. Huntington's chorea
8. Metabolic lesions
    a. Hyperglycaemia
    b. Wernicke's encephalopathy
    c. Wilson's disease
9. Drug-induced
    a. Tricyclic antidepressants
    b. Phenytoin
    c. Phenothiazines
10. Pseudogaze palsies
    a. Myasthenia gravis
    b. Chronic progressive external ophthalmoplegia

thyroid,

VERTICAL GAZE PALSIES

1. Focal midbrain disease, e.g. Parinaud's syndrome
2. Basal ganglia disease, e.g. Steele-Richardson syndrome, kernicterus *PSP*
3. Metabolic disease, e.g. Maple syrup disease, Wernicke's encephalopathy
4. Drug-induced
5. Pseudogaze palsies

Internuclear ophthalmoplegia
1. Features
    a. Lesion in medial longitudinal fasciculus
    b. Limitation of adduction of one eye *ipsilateral to INO*
    c. Ataxic nystagmus in abducting eye *contralateral eye away from INO*
    d. Unilateral or bilateral
    e. Symmetrical or asymmetrical
    f. Convergence usually good
    g. Diplopia not always present
2. Causes
    a. Multiple sclerosis
    b. Arteriosclerosis
    c. Tumours (gliomas)

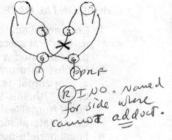

R INO - Named for side where cannot adduct.

'One and a half' syndrome
1. Features
    a. Unilateral pontine lesion
    b. Affects horizontal gaze centre and medial longitudinal fasciculus
    c. Ipsilateral gaze palsy and internuclear ophthalmoplegia
    d. Only movement is abduction of contralateral eye (with ataxic nystagmus)

2. Causes
   a. Multiple sclerosis
   b. Basilar artery occlusion
   c. Pontine metastasis

OCULAR MANIFESTATIONS OF BASAL GANGLIA DISEASE

1. Parkinson's disease
   a. Seborrhoeic blepharitis
   b. Reduced blinking
   c. Reduced saccades (hypometric)
   d. Reduced glabellar reflex suppression
   e. Blepharospasm
   f. Oculogyric crisis (especially drug-induced)
2. Steele-Richardson syndrome   *PSP! - death in 5 years: dementia*
   a. Decreased saccades (vertical early, horizontal later)
   b. Progressive vertical and horizontal gaze palsy
   c. Spasm of fixation
3. Wilson's disease
   a. Sunflower cataract
   b. Kayser-Fleischer ring in cornea
   c. Ocular movements not affected
4. Kernicterus
   Progressive loss of eye movement, especially upgaze

HEADACHE AND FACIAL PAIN

1. Acute
   a. Subarachnoid haemorrhage
   b. Meningitis/encephalitis
   c. Focal inflammation of scalp
   d. Sinusitis
   e. Dental infection
   f. Acute uveitis
   g. Acute glaucoma
   h. Scleritis
   i. Herpes zoster
   j. Cervical spondylitis
   k. Giant cell arteritis
   l. Trauma
2. Recurrent
   a. Migraine
   b. Cluster headaches
   c. Asthenopia
   d. Cerebral aneurysm or angioma
   e. Hypertensive headache (severe hypertension)

3. Chronic
   a. Muscle tension
   b. Depression
   c. Cerebral tumour
   d. Pituitary or nasopharyngeal tumour
   e. Paget's disease
   f. Post traumatic
   g. Raised intracranial pressure
   h. Chronic subdural haemorrhage
   i. Post herpetic neuralgia
   j. Trigeminal neuralgia
   k. Costen's syndrome (temporomandibular osteoarthritis)

MIGRAINE

1. Common migraine
   a. Any age. Males = Females
   b. Little or no prodrome
   c. Throbbing headache
   d. Photophobia
   e. Nausea
   f. Seclusion sought
   g. Pallor
2. Classic migraine
   a. Any age. Males = Females
   b. Less severe when older
   c. Trigger factors
   d. Visual prodrome, e.g. fortification spectra
   e. Intense headache (unilateral)
   f. Photophobia
   g. Nausea
   h. Seclusion sought
   i. Pallor
3. Complicated migraine
   a. Hemiplegic or hemiparetic
   b. Ophthalmoplegic
   c. Retinal
   d. Basilar
   e. Abdominal
   f. Oculosympathetic
4. Childhood migraine
   a. Brief attacks
   b. Pallor, nausea, vomiting
   c. Usually no headaches

NYSTAGMUS

Defect of ocular posture control

Types: 1. Pendular (associated with poor vision)
2. Jerk (associated with CNS disease)
3. Horizontal or vertical
4. Oblique
5. Rotary
6. Mixed

or

1. Physiological
   a. Optokinetic
   b. Vestibular
   c. Endpoint
2. Vestibular
   a. Lesion in inner ear, 8th nerve, brainstem/vestibular pathways
   b. Jerk, present in primary position of gaze but usually lessens on fixation
   c. Can have associated vertigo
3. Gaze-evoked
   a. Jerk, not present in primary position of gaze
   b. Main causes — drugs (anticonvulsants, major tranquillizers)
   c. Main causes — brainstem/cerebellar lesions
4. Motor imbalance
   a. Congenital nystagmus — pendular or jerk
      — X-linked or autosomal dominant
      — binocular, usually horizontal
      — damps with convergence
      — may nod or have compensatory head posture
      — vision may be normal
   b. Latent nystagmus — in dissociated vertical deviation
   c. Ataxic nystagmus — in internuclear ophthalmoplegia
   d. Spasmus nutans — infantile pendular nystagmus
      — compensatory head posture and head nodding
      — resolves by the age of three
   e. Periodic alternating nystagmus — in brainstem disease (usually disseminated sclerosis or vascular)
   f. Downbeat nystagmus — foramen magnum lesions
   g. Upbeat nystagmus — drug toxicity, e.g. anticonvulsants
      — posterior fossa lesions
   h. Convergence-retraction nystagmus — in dorsal midbrain syndrome, e.g. Parinaud's
   i. See-saw nystagmus — chiasmal lesions

5. Sensory deprivation
   a. Pendular
   b. Causes — congenital or early onset cataracts
                 — macular or optic nerve hypoplasia
                 — albinism
                 — Leber's congenital amaurosis
                 — congenital glaucoma

Causes of external ophthalmoplegia
1. 3rd, 4th and 5th nerve palsies
2. Thyroid ophthalmopathy
3. Orbital trauma
4. Orbital tumour
5. Orbital cellulitis
6. Myopathies
7. Myasthenia gravis
8. Special oculomotility syndromes, e.g. Duane's syndrome
9. Myositis

Myasthenia gravis
1. Features
   a. Autoimmune abnormality at neuromuscular junctions
   b. Antiacetylcholine receptor antibodies (IgG)
   c. Females > Males
   d. Average age of onset 15–50 years
   e. 75% present with ocular features
   f. Increasing fatigue on exercise
   g. Variable muscle weakness
   h. Dysarthria, dysphagia
   i. Facial weakness ('snarl')
   j. Respiratory failure
   k. Variable ptosis
   l. Variable ophthalmoplegia
2. Associations
   a. Penicillamine treatment
   b. Rheumatoid arthritis
   c. Systemic lupus erythematosus
   d. Thyrotoxicosis
   e. Thymic hyperplasia or tumour
3. Treatment
   a. Anticholinesterases
   b. Steroids
   c. Thymectomy
   d. Plasmapheresis
   e. Immunosuppressive drugs
   f. Conservative ocular treatment, e.g. ptosis crutches

Medical ophthalmology

ARTHRITIDES AND CONNECTIVE TISSUE DISEASES

Rheumatoid arthritis
A chronic systemic inflammatory condition characterized by a persistent, peripheral, symmetrical polyarthritis. Common disease. Females > Males
1. General features
   a. Arthritis — symmetrical and predominately peripheral
   b. Nodules — on pressure points, tendons and internal organs
   c. Vascular
      (i) Raynaud's phenomenon
      (ii) Splinter haemorrhages in nail folds
      (iii) Necrotizing arteritis affecting digits and occasionally internal organs
      (iv) Skin ulceration
      (v) Occasionally organ infarction
   d. Lung — nodules and fibrosis
   e. Heart — pericarditis
   f. Neuromuscular
      (i) Proximal myopathy and sensory neuropathy
      (ii) Atlanto-axial subluxation may result in spinal cord compression
   g. Kidneys — amyloidosis
2. Ocular features
   a. Keratoconjunctivitis sicca
   b. Cornea
      (i) Keratitis
      (ii) Peripheral corneal thinning ('contact lens' cornea). If very severe may perforate
   c. Episcleritis
   d. Scleritis

Systemic lupus erythematosus
Multisystem autoimmune condition characterized by autoantibodies to double-stranded DNA. Females > Males
1. General features
   a. Joints — Migratory symmetrical polyarthralgia
   b. Skin
      (i) Facial butterfly rash
      (ii) Photosensitivity
      (iii) Discoid rash
      (iv) Nailfold infarcts
      (v) Raynaud's phenomenon
   c. Kidneys — antigen-antibody complex deposition which may result in proteinuria, nephritic syndrome or chronic renal failure with hypertension
   d. Lungs — pleurisy
   e. Heart — pericarditis
   f. Nervous system
      (i) Peripheral neuropathy
      (ii) Psychosis
2. Ocular features
   a. Eyelid erythema with facial butterfly rash
   b. Telangiectasia
   c. Keratoconjunctivitis sicca
   d. Keratitis with peripheral corneal thinning
   e. Scleritis
   f. Retinopathy
      (i) 'Primary'. Retinal vasculitis with cotton wool spots. Disc oedema and haemorrhages
      (ii) 'Secondary' to hypertension

Scleroderma
Chronic disease dominated by cutaneous manifestations.
Females > Males
1. General features
   a. Skin
      (i) Raynaud's phenomenon
      (ii) Tight skin with swelling in early stages
      (iii) 'Purse-string mouth'
      (iv) Nail-fold infarcts
      (v) Calcinosis
   b. Bowel — oesophageal and small intestine fibrosis causing dysphagia and malabsorption
   c. Lungs — fibrosis
   d. Heart — myocarditis and pericarditis
   e. Kidneys — hypertension and renal failure
   f. Musculoskeletal — polyarthralgia and myositis

2. Ocular features
   a. Tight skin over eyelids causing punctal ectropion and epiphora
   b. Lagophthalmos
   c. Keratoconjunctivitis sicca
   d. Iris changes suggestive of atrophy
   e. Retinopathy usually due to renal hypertension

Polymyositis and dermatomyositis
Rare. Females > Males
1. General features
   a. Muscular system
      (i) Girdle weakness (shoulder and hip)
      (ii) Muscle pain and weakness
      (iii) Dysphagia and dysphonia from laryngeal and pharyngeal muscle involvement
   b. Skin
      (i) Purple 'heliotrope' rash
      (ii) Violet oedematous lesions over small joints of hands
      (iii) Nail-fold infarcts
      (iv) Telangiectasia
      (v) Raynaud's phenomena
   c. Joints — transient arthralgia
   d. Heart — cardiomyopathy
   e. Lungs — fibrosis
2. Ocular features
   a. A heliotrope (purple) rash over the eyelids
   b. Periorbital oedema
   c. Retinopathy with cotton wool spots
   d. Diplopia due to ocular myopathy

VASCULITIDES

Giant cell arteritis
Arteritis affecting medium and large muscular arteries. Patients rarely less than 60 years old. Females > Males
1. General features
   a. Fever, malaise, anorexia and weight loss
   b. Headaches
   c. Tender temporal arteries. Scalp ulceration may occur
   d. Jaw claudication or pain in tongue on eating
   e. Arteritis
      (i) Aortitis
      (ii) Bowel infarction
      (iii) Myocardial infarction
      (iv) Cerebral infarction
   f. Musculoskeletal — muscle weakness and pain, arthralgia

g. Polymyalgia rheumatica syndrome — main feature is proximal limb girdle weakness and pain
2. Ocular features
   a. Ischaemic optic neuropathy due to occlusion of posterior ciliary arteries
   b. Less commonly, central retinal artery occlusion
   c. Ocular palsies due to muscle or nerve ischaemia
   d. Cortical blindness
   e. Anterior segment ischaemia
3. Histology
   a. Artery wall thickened by inflammatory cells (histiocytes, lymphocytes and giant cells)
   b. Reaction directed against medial muscle cells and internal elastic lamina
   c. Vascular lumen narrowed by fibroblastic proliferation in lumen. May be occluded by thrombus

Polyarteritis nodosa
Systemic vasculitis affecting medium-sized and small arteries.
Males > Females
1. General features
   a. Kidney
      (i) Hypertension which may be malignant
      (ii) Nephritic or nephrotic syndrome
      (iii) Renal failure
   b. Heart
      (i) Myocardial infarction
      (ii) Angina
      (iii) Pericarditis
   c. Bowel — pain and infarction
   d. Skin — arteritic lesions
   e. Joints — arthritis
   f. Nervous system — peripheral neuropathy
2. Ocular features
   a. Necrotizing sclerokeratitis
   b. Retinopathy
      (i) 'Primary' vasculitis with occlusion
      (ii) 'Secondary' due to hypertension
   c. Yellow choroidal foci
   d. Ischaemic optic neuropathy
   e. Transient focal detachments
   f. Rarely aneurysms of retinal vessels

Wegner's granulomatosis
1. General features
   Necrotizing vasculitis with involvement of:
   a. Upper respiratory tract — haemoptysis

   b. Kidneys (renal failure major cause of death)
   c. Skin lesions
   In addition, pyrexia, weight loss, peripheral neuropathy and
   cerebral vasculitis
2. Ocular features
   a. Non-specific conjunctivitis with subconjunctival
      haemorrhages
   b. Episcleritis
   c. Scleritis
   d. Corneal infiltration and ulceration
   e. Nasolacrimal duct obstruction
   f. Orbital involvement — proptosis, painful ophthalmoplegia,
      chemosis, retinal venous congestion and optic nerve
      involvement
   g. Retinopathy — arterial narrowing, venous tortuosity, cotton
      wool spots, choroidal thickening, cystoid macular oedema
      and choroidoretinitis

Sjögren's syndrome
Chronic inflammatory autoimmune disorder characterized by a
mixed cellular infiltration of exocrine glands, notably the lacrimal
and salivary glands
1. Features
   a. Dry eyes (xerophthalmia)
   b. Dry mouth (xerostomia)
   c. Dyspareunia and chest infections
2. Types
   a. Primary Sjögren's syndrome
      (i)   The 'sicca' complex with no associated disease
      (ii) Hypergammaglobulinaemia 50%
      (iii) Rheumatoid factor 80%
      (iv) Antinuclear factor 80%
      (v)   Other autoantibodies (salivary gland, gastric parietal
            cell and smooth muscle)
      (vi) Cryoglobulinaemia
   b. Secondary Sjögren's syndrome
      Associated with a connective tissue disease
3. Associations
   a. Rheumatoid arthritis
   b. Systemic lupus erythematosus
   c. Polymyositis/dermatomyositis
   d. Scleroderma
   e. Polyarteritis nodosa
   f. Graves' disease
   g. Chronic active hepatitis and primary biliary cirrhosis
   h. Myasthenia gravis
   i. Coeliac disease

    j. Mixed connective tissue disease
    k. Non-Hodgkins lymphoma. Risk increased 40 times in
       Sjögren's syndrome
4. Pathology — inflammation and infiltration by plasma cells and
   lymphocytes with subsequent fibrosis
5. Management
    a. Treat associated conditions
    b. Tear replacement
    c. Topical mucolytic agent
    d. Vaginal lubricants

AIDS (ACQUIRED IMMUNE DEFICIENCY SYNDROME)

1. Definition
   The diagnosis is made in people who have both
    a. A reliably diagnosed disease that is at least moderately
      indicative of underlying cellular immune deficiency, e.g.
      Kaposi's sarcoma or *Pneumocystis carinii* pneumonia
    b. No other known underlying cause of cellular immune
      deficiency
2. Causal agent
   Human immunodeficiency virus (HIV). Also known as Human T
   cell lymphotropic virus (HTLV-III) and lymphadenopathy-
   associated virus (LAV)
3. Clinical states after HIV infection
    a. Acquired immune deficiency syndrome
    b. Aids related complex (ARC)
      People with two or more symptoms or signs of specific,
      chronic unexplained conditions for three months or longer,
      together with two or more abnormal laboratory values
      (i) Signs and symptoms — pyrexia of more than two
         months, chronic diarrhoea, weight loss of 10% body
         weight, malaise and lethargy, persistent generalized
         lymphadenopathy, hepatosplenomegaly, hairy
         leukoplakia or minor oral infections
      (ii) Laboratory findings — HIV antibodies or virus isolation,
         lymphopaenia, leucopaenia, anaemia,
         thrombocytopaenia, raised ESR, immunoglobulin or
         immunological abnormalities
    c. Persistent generalized lymphadenopathy (PGL)
      Unexplained lymphadenopathy in at least two extra-
      inguinal sites for more than three months
    d. Asymptomatic carriers of the virus
4. Prognosis
    a. AIDS is universally fatal. Life expectancy depends on
      presenting disease, e.g. Kaposi's sarcoma alone carries a
      mean survival of 125 weeks as opposed to *Pneumocystis
      carinii* where mean survival is 35 weeks

    b. 60% of infected individuals remain asymptomatic carriers, 33% develop PGL or ARC and the remaining 7% develop AIDS within 3 years
5. Transmission (UK 1986)
    a. Homosexuals/bisexuals 89%
    b. Recipients of blood products 5.5%
    c. Association with Africa 3%
    d. Intravenous drug users 1%
    e. Heterosexual contacts 1%
    f. Unknown 0.5%
6. General features
    a. Pulmonary
       (i) Infectious — *Pneumocystis carinii*, cytomegalovirus, *Mycobacterium avium, cryptococcus neoformans, Mycobacterium tuberculosis*
      (ii) Non-infectious — Kaposi's sarcoma, non-specific pneumonitis, adult respiratory distress syndrome
    b. Skin
       (i) Infectious — herpes zoster and simplex, warts, candidiasis and other fungal infections
      (ii) Non-infectious — Kaposi's sarcoma, immune complex vasculitis, thrombocytopenic purpura, hairy leukoplakia and seborrhoeic dermatitis
    c. Gastrointestinal — Kaposi's sarcoma, cytomegalovirus, *Cryptosporidium*, shigellosis, salmonellosis, Campylobacter, *Entamoeba histolytica, Giardia lamblia*, candidiasis, herpes simplex
    d. CNS
       (i) Cytomegalovirus — meningo-encephalitis
      (ii) *Toxoplasma gondii* — mass lesions
      (iii) *Cryptococcus neoformans* — relapsing subacute meningitis
      (iv) CNS lymphomas — mass lesions
      (v) Papovaviruses — diffuse subacute brain disease
      (vi) Herpes simplex virus — encephalomyelitis
     (vii) HIV encephalopathy — progressive dementia
7. Ocular features
    a. Conjunctival Kaposi sarcoma
    b. Keratitis
    c. Episcleritis
    d. Uveitis
    e. Retinal oedema and haemorrhages
    f. Cotton wool spots (even occurring on their own indicate a poor prognosis)
    g. Flame-shaped haemorrhages
    h. Retinal vascular sheathing
    i. Choroidal granulomas
    j. Secondary cytomegalovirus retinitis
    k. Papillitis

Infectious mononucleosis (glandular fever)
Caused by the Epstein-Barr virus
1. General features
    a. Fever and malaise
    b. Pharyngitis with palatal petechiae and tonsillar exudate
    c. Cervical lymphadenopathy and hepatosplenomegaly
    d. Arthralgia
    e. Macular-papular rash (especially if ampicillin given)
2. Ocular features
    a. Oedema of eyelids and periorbital tissues
    b. Conjunctivitis (follicular or membranous)
    c. Subconjunctival haemorrhages

BLOOD DISORDERS

Ocular features of any anaemia
1. Pale conjunctiva
2. Retinal haemorrhages
3. Retinal haemorrhages with white centres (Roth's spots)

Causes of Roth's spots
1. Anaemia
2. Subacute bacterial endocarditis ← ←←
3. Leukaemia
4. Hypertension
5. Diabetes   candida

Leukaemias
Ocular features
1. Orbital involvement (one of the commoner causes of proptosis in children)
2. Lid haemorrhage
3. Iris involvement with hypopyon or hyphaema
4. Vitreous infiltration (rare)
5. Retinal neovascularization
6. Leukaemic retinopathy with retinal haemorrhages, Roth's spots and tortuous dilated veins
7. Cotton wool spots
8. Optic nerve head infiltration
9. Papilloedema due to raised intracranial pressure from CNS infiltration

Myeloma
Ocular features
1. Corneal crystalline deposits
2. Conjunctival vessel sludging
3. Retinal vascular tortuosity and haemorrhages

4. 'Sausage-link' retinal veins, particularly in Waldenström's macroglobulinaemia (IgM myeloma)
5. Cotton-wool spots
6. Uveal effusion
7. Optic disc swelling

SKIN DISORDERS

Pseudoxanthoma elasticum (PXE)
Autosomal recessive
1. General features
   a. Skin changes on neck, axilla, antecubital fossa and paraumbilical region ('chicken skin')
   b. Vascular
      (i) Weak pulses
      (ii) Calcification
      (iii) Intermittent claudication
      (iv) Angina
   c. Gastrointestinal — bleeding
2. Ocular features
   a. Angioid streaks and PXE = Grönblad–Strandberg syndrome
   b. Pigmentary retinal mottling (peau d'orange)
   c. Peripapillary choroidal atrophy
   d. Drusen at the optic nerve head

Atopic eczema
Ocular features
   a. Chronic keratoconjunctivitis
   b. Keratoconus
   c. Giant papillary conjunctivitis
   d. Cataracts

Acne rosacea
1. General features
   a. Telangiectasia, pustules and papules
   b. Hypertrophic sebaceous glands
   c. Rhinophyma
   d. 4th to 6th decades
2. Ocular features
   a. Keratitis with peripheral vascularization and thinning of the cornea. Occasionally thinned areas may perforate. Scarring and pannus may obscure vision
   b. Blepharoconjunctivitis
   c. Recurrent chalazia
   d. Episcleritis

PHAKOMATOSES

A group of disorders in which neurological abnormalities are combined with congenital defects of skin, retina and other organs

Sturge-Weber syndrome
Not inherited
Features
- a. Cutaneous angioma over the first and second divisions of trigeminal nerve
- b. Associated meningeal angioma which may cause focal epilepsy. Intracranial calcification of the angioma may occur
- c. Glaucoma in 50%
- d. Cavernous haemangioma of the choroid

Neurofibromatosis
Autosomal dominant. Prevalence — at least 1 in 5000 population
1. General features
   - a. Café au lait spots.
     - (i) In children > 6 café au lait spots > than 0.5 cm in diameter
     - (ii) In adults, > 6 café au lait spots > 1.5 cm in diameter
   - b. Cutaneous neurofibromas
   - c. Axillary freckling (unique to neurofibromatosis)
   - d. 25% have neurological complications including
     - (i) Plexiform neuromas
     - (ii) Tumours of the CNS
     - (iii) Mental handicap
     - (iv) Epilepsy
   - e. Congenital bone defects
   - f. Endocrine tumours, e.g. phaeochromocytoma
   - g. Scoliosis
2. Ocular features
   - a. Eyelid plexiform neuroma
   - b. Iris nodules (Lisch nodules) (95%). Confirms diagnosis if café au lait spots are also present
   - c. Prominent corneal nerves (6%)
   - d. Glaucoma
   - e. Choroidal naevi
   - f. Astrocytic hamartomas (29%)   *Neurilemma*
   - g. Optic nerve gliomas and orbital tumours. Also glial tissue overlying optic disc
   - h. Spheno-orbital encephalocele (pulsatile proptosis)
3. Types
   - a. von Recklinghausen (peripheral) neurofibromatosis (90%). Major defining features are multiple café au lait spots, peripheral neurofibromas and Lisch nodules. 30% develop one or more complications

b. Bilateral acoustic (central) neurofibromatosis. Main features
are bilateral acoustic neuromas and other nervous system
tumours, particularly meningiomas

Tuberous sclerosis
Autosomal dominant. 50% new mutations
1. General features
   a. Mental retardation
   b. Epilepsy
   c. CNS hamartomas
   d. Adenoma sebaceum
   e. Hypopigmented patches (ash leaf patches) more prominent
      under ultraviolet light
   f. Café au lait spots
   g. Shagreen patches on skin (fibrous thickenings)
   h. Subungual fibromas
2. Ocular features
   a. Hypopigmented iris spots
   b. Retinal hamartomas 50% ('mulberry' tumours when
      calcified)
   c. Papilloedema secondary to gliomas
   d. 6th nerve palsy secondary to raised intracranial pressure

von Hippel-Lindau syndrome
Autosomal dominant. Possibly on chromosome 3
1. General features
   a. Haemangioblastomas of
      (i) Cerebellum
      (ii) Medulla   with or without secondary
      (iii) Pons   polycythaemia
      (iv) Spinal cord
   b. Visceral cysts
   c. Phaeochromocytoma
   d. Hypernephroma
2. Ocular features (50%)
   a. Retinal and disc angiomas
   b. Vitreous haemorrhage
   c. Hard exudates when angioma leaks
   d. Hypertensive retinopathy if associated with
      phaeochromocytoma
   e. Papilloedema in presence of raised intracranial pressure

MISCELLANEOUS CONDITIONS

Down's syndrome
Due to trisomy or translocation of chromosome 21. Incidence — 1 in every 1800 live births
1. General features
   a. Short stature
   b. Poorly developed bridge of nose
   c. Enlarged, fissured tongue
   d. Short fingers, curved inward (clinodactyly)
   e. Broad hands with single palmar crease
   f. Heart lesions (septal defects)
2. Ocular features
   a. Hypertelorism
   b. Epicanthic folds with mongoloid slant of eyelids
   c. Ectropion
   d. Blepharoconjunctivitis
   e. Strabismus and nystagmus
   f. Keratoconus sometimes presenting with acute hydrops
   g. Brushfield's spots on iris
   h. Cataracts
   i. Abnormal retinal hypoplastic disc
   j. Refractive errors (mostly myopic)

Wilson's disease
Disease characterized by the widespread deposition of copper in tissues in association with a deficiency of alpha-2-globulin. May present with neurological or hepatic signs and symptoms
1. General features
   a. CNS
      (i) Flapping tremor wrists and shoulders
      (ii) Mental changes
      (iii) Spasticity, dysarthria and dysphagia
   b. Hepatic
      (i) Hepatosplenomegaly and jaundice
      (ii) Cirrhosis and associated symptoms and signs
2. Ocular features
   a. Kayser-Fleischer Ring — greenish-brown ring at level of Descemet's membrane
   b. 'Sunflower cataract' — central green lens opacity with tapering extensions

Gout
Clinical manifestation of sustained hyperuricaemia. Males > Females
1. General features
   a. Inflammation in a joint (classically metatarsophalangeal joint of big toe but may affect other joints)
   b. Tophi within joints, pinnae and Achilles tendon

2. Ocular features
   a. Conjunctivitis
   b. Episcleritis
   c. Scleritis
   d. Band keratopathy
   e. Urate deposits in cornea, sclera, lens, tarsus and extraocular muscle tendons

Hyperlipidaemia
Conditions associated with raised levels of plasma cholesterol and triglyceride
1. Causes
   a. Primary, e.g. familial hypercholesterolaemia
   b. Secondary, e.g. diabetes mellitus, excess alcohol intake and hypothyroidism
2. General features
   a. Xanthomas
      (i) Extensor tendons (hands)
      (ii) Achilles tendons
      (iii) Patella tendons
      (iv) Palmar
      (v) Eruptive
   b. Accelerated vascular disease
      (i) Angina
      (ii) Myocardial infarction
      (iii) Intermittent claudication
   c. Pancreatitis and abdominal pain (hypertriglyceridaemia)
3. Ocular features
   a. Xanthelasmata
   b. Arcus
   c. Lipaemia retinalis

Osteogenesis imperfecta
1. General features
   a. Skeletal
      (i) Fragile bones which fracture easily
      (ii) Short and often deformed extremities
      (iii) Chest and skull deformities
   b. Ears — hearing impairment from otosclerosis
   c. Joints — flexible, tendons may rupture
   d. Skin — thin, easily bruised
   e. Heart — mitral and aortic valve prolapse
2. Ocular features
   a. Blue sclera
   b. Keratoconus, megalocornea
   c. Cataracts
   d. 'Saturn ring' — whitening of perilimbal sclera due to lack of pigmented uvea behind sclera

Table 7 Some diseases associated with particular HLA types

HLA	Diseases	Relative risk (Normal population = 1)
HLA-B27	Ankylosing spondylitis	90
HLA-B27	Nonspecific urethritis with arthritis	25
HLA-B27	Acute anterior uveitis	13
HLA-B27	Psoriatic arthritis	4
HLA-B5	Behçet's disease	6
HLA-B7 or-DR2	Multiple sclerosis	4
HLA-DW6	Psoriasis	13
HLA-DR3	Sjögren's disease	19
HLA-DR3	Systemic lupus erythematosus	6
HLA-DR3	Graves' disease	5
HLA-DR3	Juvenile onset diabetes mellitus	4
HLA-DR3	Myasthenia gravis	3
HLA-DR4	Juvenile onset diabetes mellitus	4
HLA-DR4	Rheumatoid arthritis	4

HLA-A9 Birdshot

Pharmacology

METHODS OF DELIVERING OCULAR TREATMENT

1. Drops
   a. Achieve a high concentration
   b. Quickly washed away. After 5 minutes > 80% has entered the lacrimal drainage system
   c. Convenient for daytime use as cause minimal blurring of vision
2. Ointment
   a. Longer contact time
   b. Lower drug concentration in tears
   c. Longer shelf life than drops
   d. Cause blurring of vision
3. Gels
   a. Prolong contact time
   b. Newer gels may cause less blurring than ointment
4. Soft contact lenses
   a. Absorb drugs (small molecules) when soaked in drug
   b. Deliver high concentrations over about 4 hours. N.B. Normal soft lenses also absorb drugs
5. Membrane delivery
   a. Relatively constant rate of drug delivery reducing side-effects, e.g. 'Ocuserts' resulting in less accommodative spasm and less fluctuation in intraocular pressure
   b. Deliver drug over a longer period
   c. Useful for patients with poor compliance, but easily lost
6. Sub-conjunctival
   a. Achieves high local concentration
   b. Can be painful, particularly with antibiotics. Adequate oral analgesia and topical anaesthesia must be used
   c. May cause scarring
7. Systemic — ocular penetration variable

Factors affecting penetration of topical treatment
1. Concentration
2. Viscosity
   The higher the viscosity the longer the corneal contact time.
   Ointment and gels may increase contact time and slow drug
   release. However, there is a lower concentration achieved in
   the tears compared to drops
3. Lipid solubility
   The cornea is a fat-water-fat sandwich. Un-ionized compounds
   are lipid soluble and are thus carried across the epithelium and
   endothelium. Changing the pH may change the amount of un-
   ionized chemical, but this causes more ocular discomfort and
   damage
4. Epithelial barrier
   Removal or inflammation of the epithelium improves intraocular
   penetration of topical medications

Factors affecting ocular penetration of systemic medications
1. Blood/eye barrier — may break down in the inflamed eye
2. Protein binding — reduces amount of free drug available to
   tissues
3. Lipid solubility — better penetration with higher lipid solubility
4. Peak serum levels — higher peak concentrations result in
   greater ocular penetration
5. Low molecular weight — low molecular weight molecules
   penetrate more easily. Most antibiotics are large molecules

Table 8 The ocular autonomic system

	Sympathetic action	Parasympathetic action	Dominant receptor
Dilator pupillae	Contraction (mydriasis)	Slight relaxation	Alpha (sympathetic)
Sphincter pupillae	Slight relaxation	Contraction (miosis)	Muscarinic (parasympathetic)
Ciliary muscle	Relaxation (distance vision)	Contraction (near vision)	Muscarinic (parasympathetic)
Ciliary epithelium	Aqueous secretion	—	Beta (sympathetic)
Lacrimal gland	Slight vasoconstriction	Tear secretion	Muscarinic (parasympathetic)
Smooth muscle of lid	Contraction	—	Alpha (sympathetic)

SYMPATHETIC SYSTEM AGONISTS

1. Adrenaline (0.5–1.0%) EPI naphmine (Epiprine)
   a. Actions
      (i) Alpha and beta receptor stimulation
      (ii) Increases aqueous production
      (iii) Increases rate of aqueous outflow
      (iv) Mydriasis
      (v) Vasoconstriction
   b. Clinical uses
      (i) Open angle glaucoma
      (ii) Local vasoconstriction during surgery
      (iii) Delayed absorption of local anaesthetic
      (iv) Keeping pupil dilated during intraocular surgery
      (v) Reduction of tear secretion
      (vi) Pharmacological test in Horner's syndrome
   c. Side-effects
      (i) Irritation
      (ii) Watering
      (iii) Reactive hyperaemia
      (iv) Allergy
      (v) Blurring of vision (mydriasis)
      (vi) Black adrenochrome deposits in conjunctiva, cornea
           and contact lenses
      (vii) Cystoid macular oedema in aphakic patients (both
            intracapsular and extracapsular). Reversible
      (viii) Precipitation of acute angle closure glaucoma
      (ix) Conjunctival fibrosis
      (x) Systemic side-effects — hypertension, cardiac
          arrhythmias, headaches
2. Dipivefrin (0.1%) propine .
   a. Actions
      (i) Requires conversion by tissue enzymes to adrenaline
          (these enzymes are inactivated by anticholinesterase)
      (ii) Much greater corneal penetration than adrenaline
           (×17)
   b. Clinical uses — similar to adrenaline
   c. Side effects — similar to adrenaline but much less marked
      because pro-drug not active until activated in tissues
3. Phenylephrine (2.5% and 10%)
   a. Actions
      (i) Alpha receptor stimulation
      (ii) Causes pupil dilatation without cycloplegia
   b. Clinical uses
      (i) Mydriasis for fundal examination
      (ii) Ptosis in Horner's syndrome
      (iii) Senile ptosis
      (iv) Reduction of miotic induced iris cysts

   c. Side-effects
      (i) Pigment release into anterior chamber
      (ii) Can cause clouding of the cornea
      (iii) May precipitate angle closure glaucoma
      (iv) Blurring of vision (mydriasis)
      (v) Cardiovascular side-effects — hypertension, bradycardia
   d. Reversed by thymoxamine
4. Cocaine (2% and 4%)
   a. Actions
      (i) Stabilizes nerve cell membranes preventing passage of ions and hence electrical conduction of 'pain' impulses
      (ii) Prevents re-uptake of noradrenaline by nerve terminals
   b. Clinical uses
      (i) Very effective local anaesthetic
      (ii) Potentiates action of adrenaline. Adrenaline also prolongs local anaesthetic action of cocaine by increasing vasoconstriction
      (iii) Pharmacological test in Horner's syndrome
      (iv) Paralyses parasites on eye
      (v) Precipitates with iodine. Has been used to cauterize dendritic ulcers
   c. Side-effects
      (i) Corneal epithelial damage causing clouding of the cornea
      (ii) Dilates pupil. May precipitate angle closure glaucoma. Should not be used in procedures where a small pupil is required, e.g. corneal graft
5. Hydroxyamphetamine (1%)
   a. Action — causes release of noradrenaline from normal nerve terminal
   b. Clinical use — diagnostic test in Horner's syndrome
6. Apraclonidine (1%) *to pidine)*
   a. Action — α-adrenergic agonist
   b. Clinical use — <u>reduces intraocular pressure</u> *- post yag!!*
   c. Side-effects
      (i) Dry mouth
      (ii) Fatigue
      (iii) Lid retraction
      (iv) Mydriasis
      (v) Conjunctival blanching

SYMPATHETIC SYSTEM ANTAGONISTS

1. Timolol maleate (0.25%–0.5%)
   a. Actions
      (i) Nonselective beta$_1$ and beta$_2$ receptor blocker
      (ii) Blocks cell membrane transport systems

    (iii) Competes with adrenaline and noradrenaline for receptor sites

    (iv) Reduces aqueous secretion

    (v) Maximal action over 12 hours, but may last several weeks

b. Clinical use — open angle glaucoma

c. Side-effects

    (i) Bronchospasm

    (ii) Cardiac — arrhythmias (especially bradycardia), heart failure. These may be potentiated by cardiac suppressants such as verapamil

    (iii) CNS, e.g depression

Some other topical beta-blockers:

    Carteolol (1 and 2%) — partial agonist activity (intrinsic sympathomimetic activity). In theory keeps pulse rate from falling too low

    Betaxolol (0.5%) — cardio-selective. Mainly a $beta_1$ receptor blocker

    Levobunolol (0.25–0.5%) — non-selective beta blocker

    Metipranolol (0.1–0.5%) — non-selective beta blocker

2. Thymoxamine (0.1–0.5%)

a. Actions

    (i) Competitive alpha receptor antagonist

    (ii) Maximum effect in 30 minutes

    (iii) Lasts 2 hours

b. Clinical use — reversal of phenylephrine drops

c. Side-effects

    (i) Miosis

    (ii) Transient ptosis

3. Guanethidine (5%, also 1% and 3% and with adrenaline as 'Ganda')

a. Actions

    (i) Displaces noradrenaline from nerve terminals

    (ii) Miosis and ptosis in 30 minutes

    (iii) Maximum action 24 hours

b. Clinical uses

    (i) Lid retraction in thyrotoxicosis

    (ii) Open angle glaucoma in combination with adrenaline (1 + 0.2%, 3 + 0.5% as 'Ganda')

c. Side-effects

    (i) Miosis (initially mydriasis) ⎫

    (ii) Ptosis ⎬ Like a Horner's syndrome

    (iii) Ganda 5 + 1% withdrawn due to cicatricial conjunctival changes

PARASYMPATHETIC AGONISTS

1. Pilocarpine (0.5–6%)
   a Actions
      (i) Direct parasympathetic (muscarinic) agonist
      (ii) 30 minutes to maximum effect
      (iii) Lasts 4–6 hours
      (iv) Miosis
      (v) Ciliary muscle contraction causing increased trabecular meshwork outflow facility and increased accommodation
      (vi) Shallowing of anterior chamber
      (vii) Decreased uveoscleral outflow facility
      (viii) Decreased aqueous production
      (ix) Increased permeability of blood aqueous barrier
   b. Clinical uses
      (i) Glaucoma
      (ii) To reverse mydriasis
      (iii) Diagnosis of Adie's pupil (0.125%)
      (iv) For lice infestation of eyelashes
   c. Delivery forms
      (i) Drops
      (ii) With hypromellose to lessen stinging
      (iii) Contact lenses
      (iv) Membranes, e.g. 'Ocuserts'
      (v) Gel
   d. Side-effects
      (i) Reduced visual acuity — miosis (particularly important effects with central lens opacities)
                              — accommodation
      (ii) Reduced visual fields — miosis
      (iii) Allergy
      (iv) Iris cysts
      (v) Retinal detachment
      (vi) May precipitate pupil block glaucoma
      (vii) Pupil rigidity and posterior synechiae
      (viii) Brow ache
      (ix) Lens opacities
      (x) Punctal stenosis
      (xi) Higher concentrations (⩾ 4%) may cause cicatricial conjunctival changes
      (xii) Systemic effects — sweating
                           — nausea
                           — vomiting
                           — bradycardia
                           — diarrhoea
                           — salivation

2. Acetylcholine (1%)
   a. Actions
      (i) Direct stimulation of iris sphincter muscle
      (ii) Rapidly broken down by anticholinesterase
      (iii) Miosis lasts about 10 minutes
   b. Clinical uses — intraoperative miosis
   c. Side-effects
      (i) Transient lens opacities due to osmotic action
      (ii) Corneal oedema
      (iii) Retinal detachment
      (iv) Systemic — bradycardia
                      — hypotension
3. Methacholine (2.5%)
   a. Action — direct stimulation of parasympathetic system
   b. Clinical use — diagnosis of Adie's pupil
   c. Disadvantage — expensive
4. Carbachol (3%)
   a. Actions
      (i) Direct stimulation of parasympathetic system
      (ii) Powerful miosis
      (iii) Prolonged accommodative spasm
   b. Clinical use — chronic open angle glaucoma (in patients
      allergic to pilocarpine)
   c. Side-effects
      (i) Conjunctival toxicity
      (ii) Similar to pilocarpine
5. Physostigmine (0.2%, 0.5%)
   a. Actions
      (i) Reversible cholinesterase inhibitor
      (ii) Miosis in 10 minutes, lasts 4 hours
      (iii) Mild miosis may persist for several days
      (iv) Ciliary spasm
   b. Clinical use — glaucoma
   c. Side-effects
      (i) Similar to pilocarpine
      (ii) Eyelid twitching
      (iii) Eyelid depigmentation
6. Edrophonium (10 mg/ml injection)
   a. Actions   Indirect ·
      (i) Reversible cholinesterase inhibitor
      (ii) Improves ptosis and diplopia in myasthenia gravis for
           about 5 minutes
   b. Clinical use — diagnosis of myasthenia gravis
      Tensilon test
      (i) 10 mg of edrophonium in syringe
      (ii) Inject intravenous normosaline to check placebo effect
      (iii) Inject 1–2 mg of edrophonium and wait one minute

(iv) Only if no response inject rest of edrophonium
(v) Positive response is improvement in ophthalmoplegia or ptosis which relapses within minutes. Intraocular pressure may also rise up to 5 mmHg but this may only be unilateral
c. Side-effects
(i) Anaphylactic reaction
(ii) Cholinergic overreaction can occur in patients with myasthenia gravis after edrophonium is given. *Resuscitation equipment must be readily available*

7. Ecothiopate or Phospholine Iodide (0.06, 0.12 and 0.25%)
a. Actions
(i) Irreversible cholinesterase inhibitor
(ii) Miosis for 2–4 weeks
(iii) Ciliary spasm 7 days
(iv) Fall in intraocular pressure maximal over 24 hours
b. Clinical uses
(i) Chronic open angle glaucoma
(ii) Accommodative esotropia
c. Side-effects
(i) *Abnormal response to muscle relaxants used in general anaesthesia*
(ii) Conjunctival vasodilatation and fibrosis
(iii) Spasm of accommodation
(iv) Corneal endothelial disturbance in high dosage
(v) Iritis
(vi) Iris cyst formation
(vii) Cataract
(viii) Retinal detachment
(ix) Eyelid twitching
(x) May precipitate pupil block glaucoma
(xi) Posterior synechiae
(xii) Systemic toxicity:
CVS — bradycardia, hypertension, hypotension and sweating
CNS — nausea, vomiting, fatigue, paraesthesia, insomnia, nightmares, drowsiness, muscle twitching and coma
GI — salivation, abdominal cramp and diarrhoea

PARASYMPATHETIC ANTAGONISTS

1. Atropine (1%)
a. Actions
(i) Competitive postganglionic muscarinic receptor blockade
(ii) Causes pupillary dilatation and cycloplegia
(iii) Decreases lacrimal secretion and vascular permeability

b. Clinical uses
  (i) Uveitis — pupillary dilatation
              — cycloplegia
              — possible anti-inflammatory action
  (ii) Cycloplegic refraction — most effective cycloplegic agent
  (iii) Amblyopia (to blur vision of good eye)
  (iv) Dilatation of the pupil for fundal examination where prolonged effect is required, e.g. retinal detachment
c. Side-effects
  (i) Allergy
  (ii) Acute angle closure glaucoma (dilatation may also increase intraocular pressure in patients with chronic open angle glaucoma)
  (iii) Blurring of vision — cycloplegia
                          — increase in optical aberrations due to the mydriasis
      (Reversal of dilatation with pilocarpine may actually worsen vision in some patients)
  (iv) Systemic reactions — tachycardia
                         — facial flush *red*
                         — tremor
                         — dryness of mouth and skin *dry*
                         — delerium *crazy*
      These occur particularly in elderly and young patients. For a 4.5 kg child a lethal dose is (10 mg)(20 drops of a 1% solution)   *·5 mg / drop.*
2. Hyoscine (0.25 and 0.5%)
   Similar to atropine but shorter acting
3. Homatropine (1–2%)
   Similar to atropine but shorter acting
4. Lachesine (1%)
   Maximum mydriatic action at one hour and lasts 5–6 hours. Useful if patient allergic to atropine
5. Cyclopentolate (0.5–2%)
   Shorter acting than homatropine but better cycloplegic. Useful for short-term dilatation of pupil and cycloplegia
6. Tropicamide (0.5–1%)
   Short acting with only partial cycloplegia. Useful for short-term dilatation of the pupil
7. Combination of drug for dilatation of the pupil
   Mydricaine No 2 = atropine 1 mg, adrenaline 0.12 ml 1 in 1000 solution and procaine 6.0 mg, made up to 0.3 ml volume
   Given subconjunctivally to dilate the pupil
   Relatively large dose of atropine so caution in treating
   a. Elderly
   b. Young patients
   c. Patients who may need bilateral injections

Smaller dose ampoule available (mydricaine No 1 which has half the concentration of mydricaine No 2)

Table 9

Drug	Mydriasis		Cycloplegia	
	Max effect (minutes)	Recovery (days)	Max effect (hours)	Recovery (days)
Atropine 1%	45	10	6	14
Hyoscine(scop)¼%	35	7	1	7
Homatropine 2%	60	3	1	3
Cyclopentolate 1%	60	1	1	1
Tropicamide 1%	40	0.25	0.5	0.25

ORAL CARBONIC ANHYDRASE INHIBITORS
Acetazolamide *(Diamox)*   Methazolamide *(Neptazane)*
  a. Actions
    (i) Inhibition of carbonic anhydrase activity
    (ii) Reduces the bicarbonate in the aqueous humour and the water secreted with it
    (iii) Fall in intraocular pressure of 30–60%
    (iv) Action over 6–12 hours after oral treatment. Duration of action can be prolonged by sustained release capsules
  b. Clinical uses
    (i) Reduction of intraocular pressure
    (ii) Reduction of intracranial pressure
    (iii) 'Mountain sickness'
    (iv) Macular oedema
  c. Side-effects
    (i) Malaise
    (ii) Anorexia
    (iii) Nausea
    (iv) Depression
    (v) Parasthesiae
    (vi) Transient myopia
    (vii) Hypokalaemia
    (viii) Metabolic acidosis
    (ix) Renal stones
    (x) Deafness in patients with Meniere's disease
    – Impotence, Stevens Johnson, *Aplastic Anaemia* – agranulocytosis.

TOPICAL NONSTEROIDAL ANTI-INFLAMMATORY AGENTS
1. Flurbiprofen sodium
  a. Actions
    (i) Competes with arachidonic acid for cyclo-oxygenase binding

       (ii) Prevents arachidonic acid converting to prostaglandin
      (iii) May prevent vasodilatation, breakdown of the blood-aqueous humour barrier, intraoperative miosis and increased intraocular pressure
   b. Clinical uses
       (i) Prevention of miosis during intraocular surgery
      (ii) Reduction of ocular inflammation, e.g. scleritis
     (iii) Prevention of cystoid macular oedema
2. Sodium cromoglycate (drops 2%, ointment 4%)
   a. Actions
       (i) Inhibition of mast cell degranulation, the local release of vasoactive amines and inflammatory agents
      (ii) Stabilizes mast cell membrane and modulates the intracellular events that lead to mast cell degranulation
   b. Clinical uses
       (i) Hayfever conjunctivitis
      (ii) Recurrent allergic conjunctivitis
     (iii) Perennial allergic conjunctivitis
     (iv) Vernal keratoconjunctivitis
      (v) Giant papillary conjunctivitis
     (vi) Ligneous conjunctivitis
    (vii) Marginal corneal ulceration

Table 10 Pharmacological pupil tests

	Normal	Condition		
		Central Horner's syndrome	Postganglionic Horner's syndrome	Primary iris disease
Drops				
Adrenaline (0.1%)	No change	No change	Full dilatation	No change
Cocaine (4%)	Full dilatation	Partial dilatation	No change	No change
Hydroxy-amphetamine (1%)	Full dilatation	Full dilatation	No change	No change

Pupil tests in Horner's syndrome
1. Adrenaline (0.1%) test
   a. Relies on denervation hypersensitivity
   b. Not present immediately after sympathetic chain damage occurs
2. Cocaine (4%) test
   a. Prevents re-uptake of noradrenaline by nerve terminals of the dilator pupillae muscle
   b. Observe 30 minutes after instillation

    c. Test is dose-dependent. If there is epithelial damage (e.g. from applanation) this may enhance cocaine entry and cause spurious dilatation

3. Hydroxyamphetamine (1%) test
    a. Causes release of noradrenaline from the normal nerve terminal
    b. Observe 30 minutes after instillation, but may take up to 2 hours to work in patients with heavily pigmented irides
    c. Should not be done within two days of cocaine test as cocaine blocks the uptake of hydroxyamphetamine at nerve terminals

Other pupil diagnostic tests

1. Drug-induced pupillary dilatation
    a. Theory
       (i) Drugs which paralyse the sphincter do so by blocking the muscarinic receptor sites
       (ii) A weak pilocarpine solution cannot bind with enough receptors to cause pupillary constriction
    b. Technique
       (i) Apply 0.5% pilocarpine to each eye
       (ii) Observe after 30 minutes
    c. Positive result
    Failure of the pupil to constrict. This suggests drug-induced pupillary dilatation. A traumatic mydriasis will also be unresponsive

2. Adie's myotonic pupil
    a. Theory
       (i) Denervation hypersensitivity occurs after damage to the parasympathetic nerve supply to the pupil
       (ii) Denervation hypersensitivity is not immediately present
    b. Technique
       (i) 0.125% pilocarpine to each eye
       (ii) Observe after 20 minutes
       (iii) Methacholine 2.5% may also be used but this is expensive and has to be freshly prepared
    c. Positive result — constriction of a previously dilated pupil

SOME OCULAR SIDE-EFFECTS OF SYSTEMIC DRUGS

1. Eyelids/cornea/conjunctiva
    a. Phenothiazines, e.g. chlorpromazine. Discolouration of the skin and golden-brown granules in the conjunctiva and fine deposits in the cornea
    b. Stevens-Johnson syndrome secondary to hypersensitivity from drugs such as sulphonamides
    c. Oculomucocutaneous syndrome secondary to practolol

    d. Chloroquine. Deposition in the corneal epithelium sometimes in a whorl-like appearance (verticillata). Causes hazy vision, photophobia and haloes around lights

    e. Amiodarone. Skin photosensitivity and corneal verticillata

    f. Gold. Fine particles in the conjunctiva or cornea

2. Lens

    a. Corticosteroids. Posterior subcapsular lens opacities (and open angle glaucoma)

    b. Phenothiazines, e.g. chlorpromazine. Fine yellowish-brown granules beneath the anterior lens capsule

    c. Myopia from tetracyclines, sulphonamides, acetazolamide and antihistamines

3. Pupil

    a. Pupillary dilatation may precipitate angle closure glaucoma after treatment with atropine, antiparkinsonian agents and cyclotropic drugs

    b. Miosis. Particularly with opiates

4. Retina

    a. Chloroquine compounds. These have an affinity for melanin. Early visual complaints include blurring of vision, photophobia and flashes of light. Bilateral retinal changes start with an abnormal foveal reflex and parafoveal pigmentary disturbance. This leads to a 'bulls-eye' appearance

    b. Phenothiazines, e.g. thioridazine. Acute onset with diminution of vision, retinal oedema and hyperaemia of the optic disc. Chronic onset with a fine pigment scatter in the central area of the fundus extending peripherally. The pigment coalesces into plaques

    c. Oxygen. High oxygen concentrations are implicated in the retinopathy of prematurity

5. Optic nerve

    a. Antituberculosis drugs.

      (i) Streptomycin — xanthopsia with central scotoma

      (ii) Ethambutol — visual loss with colour vision defects especially to green

          — optic neuritis

          — greater risk of ocular toxicity with renal dysfunction

          — pyridoxine may help to protect from toxicity

    b. Chloramphenicol. Disc hyperaemic with haemorrhages and oedema. Occurs most frequently in children

    c. Tetracycline. Benign intracranial hypertension and papilloedema

    d. Digitalis. Disturbance of colour vision, usually sensation of yellow colouration (xanthopsia)

    e. Penicillamine. Optic neuritis
    f. Quinine is probably directly toxic with secondary vascular closure
    g. Clioquinol (enterovioform). Optic neuritis especially in Japanese
6. Ocular motility
    a. Carbamazepine and phenytoin. Nystagmus
    b. Streptomycin. Paralysis of eye muscles and nystagmus
    c. Phenothiazines and metoclopramide. Oculogyric crisis

Optics

LIGHT
1. Visible spectrum — 400 nm (blue) to 700 nm (red)
2. Theories of light
   a. Particle theory (Plank) — quanta of energy proportional to wavelength
   b. Wave theory (Maxwell) — energy passage through medium
      — particle vibration perpendicular to direction of wave
      — amplitude (maximal displacement)
      — wavelength (distance between symmetrical points)

Interference
1. Constructive — summation when waves in phase
2. Destructive — algebraic summation when waves out of phase, e.g. in corneal stroma, antireflective coatings

Diffraction
1. Production of secondary wavefronts after passage of light through slits or around edges
2. Resulting interference (Airy's discs) limits resolution through aperture

Polarization
1. All waves in same plane
2. Polarizing substances transmit in only one plane
3. Polarizing angle = incident angle producing polarized reflection (varies with refractive index)
4. Uses
   a. Reduction of glare
   b. Assessment of binocular vision, e.g. Titmus fly
   c. Checking of stress lines in lens manufacture

Photometry
1. Quantitative measurement of light
2. Luminous flux — total emission (lumen)
3. Luminous intensity — emission in given direction (candela)
4. Illumination — inverse square law

$$E = \frac{l.\cos i}{d^2}$$

  l = luminous intensity (candela)
  d = distance from source
  i = angle of incidence
5. Luminance — measurement of reflected light

Laws of reflection
1. Incident ray, reflected ray and normal in same plane
2. Angle of reflection equals angle of incidence

Reflection at a plane mirror
1. Image virtual
2. Image laterally transposed
3. Image distance equals object distance
4. Magnification equals unity

Reflection at a spherical surface
1. Centre of curvature (C)
2. Centre of mirror = principle point (P)
3. CP = principle axis
4. $\frac{1}{2}$ CP = principle focus (F)
5. Object distance = u
6. Image distance = v
7. Focal distance = f
8. Rays parallel to CP are reflected through F
9. Rays incident to C are reflected back along path

Mirror formula $\left(\dfrac{1}{f} \right) = \dfrac{1}{v} - \dfrac{1}{u}$

Magnification (M) $= \dfrac{\text{image size}}{\text{object size}} = \dfrac{v}{u}$

10. Uses
    a. Catoptric imagery
    b. Keratometers
    c. Placido's disc

Refraction
1. Change in direction of wavefront on traversing media of different optical densities (n_1, n_2)
2. Velocity of light varies with optical density

3. Refractive index (n) is the ratio of velocities $\frac{V_1}{V_{vacuum}}$
4. Snell's laws
   a. Incident angle (i), refracted angle (r) and normal are in the same plane
   b. Refractive index (n) $= \dfrac{\sin i}{\sin r}$ $n(\sin i) = n^2(\sin r)$
5. Refraction through a plate of glass — emergent ray is parallel to incident ray
6. Critical angle — ray emerging from optically dense medium refracted away from normal. At critical angle, ray refracted along interface. At greater angles, total internal reflection occurs
7. Dispersion — refractive index of medium varies with wavelength and results in separation of wavelengths
8. Refraction at a curved surface produces vergence

$$\text{Surface (vergence) power} = \frac{n_2 - n_1}{radius}$$

PRISMS

1. Portion of refracting surface bordered by two planes inclined at an angle α (refracting angle or apical angle)
2. Axis = bisection of refracting angle
3. Base = opposite side to refracting angle
4. Deviation (D) proportional to
   a. Refractive index
   b. Refracting angle
   c. Angle of incidence
5. Ophthalmic prisms $D = \dfrac{\alpha}{2}$
6. Prism power measured in prism dioptres. One dioptre = 1 cm deviation at 1 m
7. Image
   a. Erect
   b. Virtual
   c. Displaced to apex

Uses of prisms
1. Diagnostic
   a. Measurement of angle of strabismus objectively by prism cover test
   b. Measurement of strabismus subjectively by Maddox rod
   c. Assessment of possible diplopia after proposed strabismus surgery
   d. Measurement of fusional reserve
   e. Assessment of microtropia (4 dioptre prism test)
   f. Assessment of simulated blindness

2. Instruments
   a. Slit lamp/operating microscope
   b. Keratometer
   c. Pachymeter
   d. Applanation tonometer
3. Therapeutic
   a. Convergence insufficiency
   b. Relieve diplopia

Special prisms

1. Fresnel prism — 2 mm thick strip of plastic. Multiple prisms produce effect of single large prism with equivalent refracting angle
2. Reflecting prisms
   a. Porro — deviates light 180° and inverts image
   b. Dove — inverts image
3. Woolaston prism — two prisms of quartz (a double refractor) placed at 90°, producing two beams at a fixed angle

LENSES

1. Portion of a refracting medium bordered by two curved surfaces with a common axis
2. Total vergence depends on the power of each surface vergence and lens thickness
3. Sign convention

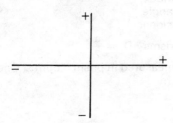

Thin lens theory

1. Ignores lens thickness
2. Optical centre of lens = nodal point (N)
3. Centres of curvature of surfaces = C_1, C_2
4. Principle axis (p) = C_1 N C_2
5. Principle foci lie on p = F_1, F_2 (F = focal point)
6. Power of lens (dioptres) = algebraic sum of vergence power. Reciprocal of P_2 (P = focal length). Positive for convex lenses, negative for concave lenses

7. Magnification

Linear $= \dfrac{\text{image size}}{\text{object size}} = \dfrac{v}{u}$

Angular $= \dfrac{\text{angle subtended by image}}{\text{angle subtended by object}}$

8. Magnification with simple loupe (assuming working distance of 25 cm)

$M = \dfrac{F}{4}$

where F = lens power (dioptres)

9. Thin lens formula $\dfrac{1}{P_2} = \dfrac{1}{v} - \dfrac{1}{u}$

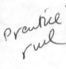

10. Prismatic effect of decentration — peripheral portions of a lens act as prisms with increasing refracting angle

$P = F \times d$

where P = prism dioptres, F = lens dioptres, d = decentration in cm

Uses — instead of actual prism addition
— up to 5 mm of displacement
— if along axis of astigmatic lens, will not affect power

Astigmatic lenses
1. Cylindrical lens
   a. Vergence power in one meridian
   b. Axis of cylinder perpendicular to power meridian
   c. Production of line image of point source, parallel to axis
2. Toric lens
   a. Cylindrical lens superimposed on spherical lens, produces blurred image within Sturm's conoid
   b. Circle of least confusion = point of maximum definition

Identification of lenses
1. Viewing through lens
   a. Direction of apparent movement of object on moving lens
      (i) Against = convex lens
      (ii) With = concave lens
   b. Apparent distortion on rotating lens = astigmatic lens
      (i) Find position of no distortion
      (ii) Check direction of apparent movement in each meridian
      (iii) Mark lens on each axis to locate optical centre
      (iv) Constant displacement = prismatic incorporation
2. Neutralization — using opposite lens power to neutralize apparent movements

3. Lens measure (e.g. Geneva) — refractive index required to calculate power
4. Focimeter
   a. Measures vertex power
   b. Measures astigmatic powers and axes
   c. Allows optical centre marking and prism assessment

Lens shape
1. Round (disadvantage of requiring lens lock or lens will rotate)
2. Round oval
3. Long oval
4. Pantoscopic (oval with flattened top)

Lens section
1. Symmetrical — simple lenses
2. Asymmetrical
   a. Best form lenses — usually meniscus-shaped to reduce aberrations

−6 D posterior curve	up to +7 D
+6 D anterior curve	up to −6 D
+1.25 D anterior curve	−6 to −10 D
Plano anterior curve	−10 to −20 D

   b. Periscopic lenses − 1.25 D base curve
   c. Aspheric lenses — flatter peripherally to reduce power and aberrations
   d. Lenticular — lens power located centrally. reduces weight and aberrations
   e. Variable focus lenses — changing lens section to increase power in down gaze

Bifocal lenses
1. Forms
   a. Franklin split = two piece
   b. Cemented ⎤
   c. Fused   ⎬ segments
   d. Solid   ⎦
2. Shape
   a. 22 or 24 mm round segments
   b. 38 or 45 mm round segments
   c. 25 or 28 mm straight top segments (D segment)
   d. Executive segments
3. Relative indications
   a. High AC/A ratio esotropia
   b. Convenience
4. Relative contraindications
   a. Anisometropia
   b. High oblique astigmatism

   c. Heterophoria
   d. Reading add more than 4 D
 5. Intolerance
   a. Related to segment size, height, power
   b. Chromatic aberration (fused segments)
   c. Prismatic jump — if insert not concentric
                     — reduced with executive and D segments
   d. Sudden changes in focal power
   e. Oblique astigmatism — near visual axis and near segment
      optical axis not coincident
   f. Muscle imbalance — due to reduced accommodative
      convergence
   g. Lack of intermediate focus

Trifocal lenses

 1. Form
   a. Intermediate power
   b. Usually $\frac{1}{2}$ power reading segment
   c. 8 mm in depth
 2. Shape
   a. D segment
   b. Executive segment

Lens aberrations (distortions in the image produced)

 1. Chromatic
   a. Related to dispersion of light
   b. Reduced by combining lenses of opposite dispersive powers
      to produce required refraction
 2. Spherical — prismatic effect of peripheral lens resulting in
   increasing deviation
   a. Reduced by
     (i) Best form lenses
     (ii) Diaphragm to exclude peripheral lens
     (iii) Lenticular lenses
     (iv) Aspheric lenses
     (v) Doublets
   b. Reduced in eye by
     (i) Peripheral corneal flattening
     (ii) Iris stop
     (iii) Different refractive index of lens nucleus and lens
        cortex
     (iv) Stiles-Crawford effect
 3. Oblique — oblique light, not parallel to principle axis. Causes
   astigmatic refraction
   a. Reduced by
     (i) Keeping incident light parallel to axis
     (ii) Diaphragm to exclude peripheral lens
     (iii) Best form lenses

b. Reduced in eye by
   (i) Aplanitic cornea
   (ii) Curved retina
   (iii) Peripheral retina has poor resolution
4. Coma — unequal magnification of object resulting from object not being on principle axis
5. Image distortion
   a. Barrel from concave lens
   b. Pincushion from convex lens
6. Curvature of field — plane object produces curved image

Thick lens theory
1. Lens thickness must be taken into account
2. Principles to simplify formulae
   a. 2 principle planes ($P_1 P_2$). Perpendicular to principle axis. Light parallel to axis incident on 1st plane is projected to focal point as if leaving from 2nd plane
   b. 2 nodal points (N_1, N_2). Points on principle axis. Light incident on N_1 leaves system as if from N_2 and parallel to the incident ray
3. True focal lengths — $P_1 F_1 = f_1$
   — $P_2 F_2 = f_2$
4. Vertex focal length — measure from lens surface to focal point
5. Back vertex power — reciprocal of vertex focal length. Different from equivalent or true power

Reduced eye (after Listing)
1. Single principle plane and nodal point
2. Distances from anterior cornea
   a. Principle plane +1.35 mm
   b. Nodal point +7.08 mm
   c. F_1 −15.70 mm
   d. F_2 +24.13 mm
   e. Lens power +15 D
   f. Aphakic power +43 D
   g. F_1 aphakic eye −21.88 mm

OPTICS OF EMMETROPIA AND AMETROPIA
1. Emmetropia — axial length equals dioptric power of eye with far point at infinity
2. States of emmetropia — as a result of appropriate matching of abnormalities far point can remain at infinity
3. Myopia — finite far point
4. Hypermetropia — virtual far point
5. Types of ametropia
   a. Axial
   b. Curvature
   c. Index

Accommodation
1. Ability of the eye to change its refractive power to maintain focus on an approaching object
2. Near point — point of nearest distinct vision
3. Range — far point to near point
4. Amplitude — change in dioptric power
5. Reducing amplitude with age a. 14 D as infant
   b. 4 D at 40 years
   c. 1 D at 60 years
6. Presbyopia — near point extends beyond reading distance reading distance usually taken as 25 cm (4 D)

Ocular astigmatism
1. Variation of refraction in different meridia
2. Regular
   Axes perpendicular
   a. With the rule
      (i) Negative cylinder horizontal

   b. Against the rule
      (i) Negative cylinder vertical

   c. Oblique
      (i) Symmetrical

      (ii) Complementary

   d. Classification
      (i) Simple — one axis ametropic
      (ii) Compound — both axes ametropic
      (iii) Mixed — each axis of opposite power

3. Bi-oblique — axes not at right angles
4. Irregular — no axes determinable
          — corneal or lenticular pathology

Optical correction of ametropia
1. Using lenses such that rays appear to come from the far point of the eye
2. If lens positioned close to the eye then far point equals focal length of the lens

Effective power
1. If lens position is altered, far point and focal point no longer coincide. Effective power of lens thus changes
2. On moving lens away from eye
   a. Positive lenses — power effectively increases
   b. Negative lenses — power effectively decreases
3. Effect of position significant if lens power is over 5 D
4. Back vertex distance = distance between the back of the lens and the corneal apex
5. Power of new lens (F_2)

$$F_2 = \frac{F_1}{1-dF_1}$$

d = distance of change in metres

Relative spectacle magnification (RSM)
1. $\text{RSM} = \dfrac{\text{corrected image size}}{\text{emmetropic image size}}$
2. Axial ametropia — RSM = 1 if correcting lens at anterior focal point
3. Index ametropia — RSM = 1 if lens at principle plane of eye
          — hypermetropia, RSM > 1 (with spectacles)
          — myopia, RSM < 1 (with spectacles). RSM tends to unity on approaching eye
4. RSM and aphakia — spectacles, RSM = 1.36
          — contact lens, RSM = 1.1
          — intraocular lens, RSM = 1.0

Anisometropia
1. Difference in refractive state between the two eyes
2. Causes
   a. Congenital, e.g. buphthalmos
   b. Acquired, e.g. nuclear sclerosis, lens dislocation and extraction
3. Hypermetropia > 1 D associated with amblyopia
4. Anisometropia > 2.50 D produces a 5% image disparity

Aniseikonia
1. Different image size in each eye
2. Measured with Goldmann eikonometer
3. Physiological aniseikonia essential for binocular single vision
4. No binocular single vision possible if there is more than a 5% disparity of image
5. Iseikonic lenses
   a. Change image size
   b. Ability relates to lens thickness and anterior curve
   c. 5% maximum change in image size
   d. Thick, heavy
   e. Difficult to manufacture
   f. Expensive

Optical problems with spectacle correction of aphakia
1. Increased image size
   a. Sensation of proximity and misjudgement of distances
   b. Patients feel small
2. Aniseikonia with unilateral aphakia
3. Prismatic effects
   a. Ring scotoma
   b. 'Jack in the box' phenomenon
4. Narrow field of vision
5. Spectacle weight and cost
6. Cosmetic

INDICATIONS FOR CONTACT LENSES
1. Optical (NHS eligibility)
   a. There must be definite improvement over spectacle corrected vision. Final decision by consultant
   b. Ametropia of 10.00 D or more
   c. Aniseikonia of 10% or more
   d. Anisometropia of 4.00 D or more
   e. Corneal irregularities — keratoconus, corneal scarring and astigmatism
   f. Therapeutic soft lenses
   g. Part of telescopic lens system
   h. Ocular pathology
      (i) Albinism
      (ii) Aniridia
      (iii) Coloboma
      (iv) Ptosis
2. Diagnostic
   a. 3 mirror, gonio and macular lenses
   b. Radio-opaque localizing lens
   c. Electrodiagnostic lenses
   d. Lens for specular microscopy

3. Occupational
   a. Sports
   b. Acting
4. Cosmetic
   a. Heterochromia
   b. Phthisis
5. Protective — shield in radiotherapy
6. Therapeutic
   a. Bandage lens — a soft, high water content lens
      (i) Bullous keratopathy
      (ii) Trichiasis
      (iii) Trauma
      (iv) Descemetocele
      (v) Prevention of erosions
      (vi) Ulcer healing
      (vii) Small leaking wound
      (viii) Filamentary keratitis
   b. Haptic lens
      (i) Prevention of symblepharon
      (ii) Ptosis, e.g. in progressive external ophthalmoplegia
   c. Soft lens soaked in drug for prolonged delivery, e.g.
      methazolamide
   d. Laser contact lens
      (i) Stabilizes eye
      (ii) Holds eyelids open
      (iii) Magnifies or provides wide angle image
      (iv) Increases convergence angle which minimizes risk of
           retinal damage, especially with Nd-YAG laser

Types of loupes
1. Hand held
2. Stand magnifier
3. Paper weight
4. Lens bars

Galilean telescope
1. Convex objective, concave eye piece
2. Separated by difference in focal length
3. Magnification $= \dfrac{\text{power of eyepiece (Fe)}}{\text{power of objective (Fo)}}$
4. Compact system
5. Erect image
6. Minimal distortion
7. May be adapted for near or distance
8. Can be spectacle mounted

9. Field of view
   a. Depends on size of objective
   b. Has an inverse relationship to magnification
   c. Increases with proximity of the system to the eye
   d. Increases as distance between lenses is reduced

Some non-optical devices for poor vision
1. Large print books
2. Good lighting
3. Large fibre tip pens
4. Large dial telephones
5. Large playing cards

Direct ophthalmoscope
1. Field of view
   a. Approximately 6°
   b. Related to
      (i) Size of sight hole — mirror
      　　　　　　　　　　　 — observer's pupil
      　　　　　　　　　　　 — subject's pupil
      (ii) State of ametropia — myopia (small field)
      　　　　　　　　　　　　 — hypermetropia (large field)
   c. Increases with proximity of ophthalmoscope to subject
2. Retinal image size
   a. Image larger in myopia
   b. Image smaller in hypermetropia
3. Magnification (simple loupe)

$$M = \frac{60}{4} = \times 15$$

Indirect ophthalmoscope
1. Field of illumination
   a. Related to state of ametropia
      (i) Myopia, large field
      (ii) Hypermetropia, smaller field
   b. Related to subject's pupil size
2. Field of view
   a. Approximately 25° field
   b. Related to
      (i) Aperture of condensing lens
      (ii) Size of observer's pupil
3. Retinal image
   a. Magnification
      (i) Using +13 D = × 5
      (ii) Using +20 D = × 3

b. Change in image size on moving lens is related to ametropic state. On moving away
   (i) Emmetropia — remains the same
   (ii) Myopia — increases
   (iii) Hypermetropia — decreases
c. Stereoscopic view
d. Ametropia has relatively little effect on image size
e. Image inverted vertically and horizontally

Measurement of corneal curvature
1. Placido's disc
2. Keratometer — measures central zone
   2 types
   a. von Helmholtz — fixed object size (O). image size (I) measured. (Rotating glass plates)
   b. Javal-Schiotz — fixed image size (I), object size (O) varied. (Mires on curved side arms)

   Corneal radius (r) $= \dfrac{2uI}{O}$

   u = focal distance of viewing telescope (constant)

Compound microscope
1. Convex objective and eyepiece
2. Separated by distance greater than focal length
3. Image inverted

Slit lamp
1. Binocular microscope coupled to projection system
2. Results in
   a. Common axis of rotation
   b. Microscope and projector having coincident foci
   c. Axis of rotation at this common point
   d. Long working distance which allows access

Slit lamp examination techniques
1. Direct focal illumination
2. Diffuse illumination
3. Retroillumination
4. Lateral illumination
5. Specular reflection
6. Sclerotic scatter
7. Blue or green filter
8. Additional techniques for fundal examination
   a. Hruby lens, −58.6 D
   b. Contact lenses, plano concave
   c. Indirect lenses, +90 D

Applanation tonometer
1. Produces image splitting to ensure standardized fluorescein ring size
2. Produced by prisms with bases in opposite directions

Pachymeter
1. For the measurement of
   a. Corneal thickness
   b. Anterior chamber depth
2. Uses Purkinje–Sanson images
   a. Image I (anterior corneal surface)
   b. Image II (posterior corneal surface)
   c. Image III (anterior lens surface)
   (Images I and II to measure corneal thickness; Images II and III to measure anterior chamber depth)
3. Types
   a. Maurice and Giardine — splits incident light
   b. Jaeger — special eyepiece

REFRACTION PROCEDURE
1. Measurement of monocular vision with and without correction
2. Cover test with and without correction
3. Measurement of interpupillary distance (IPD)
4. Place trial frame on patient and adjust IPD
5. Direct patient's gaze at distant target and carry out retinoscopy
   a. In presence of strabismus occlude fellow eye
   b. In young, fog fellow eye with plus lens
6. Subtract the reciprocal of the working distance in metres (= dioptres) from the result
7. Subjective procedure in each eye
   a. Monocular vision with retinoscopy result
   b. Check best vision sphere with Snellen test chart or duochrome
   c. Correct astigmatism with either Jackson's cross cylinder or fan and block
   d. Recheck best vision sphere (aiming for maximum plus or minimum minus)
   e. Repeat procedure for fellow eye
8. Binocular balance (to equalize accommodative state) — Humphrey, Septum, Polaroid techniques
9. Oculomotor and accommodation tests
   a. Distance heterophoria by Maddox rod
   b. Measure amplitude of accommodation, monocular and binocular. Calculate near addition. Adjust trial frame IPD
   c. Measure near heterophoria by Maddox wing
   d. Measure near point of convergence

e. Additional tests may be used if appropriate
   (i) Cover test
   (ii) Fixation disparity
   (iii) AC/A ratio
   (iv) Fusional reserves
   (v) Stereopsis
   (vi) Colour tests

RETINOSCOPY

1. Small proportion of light entering eye is reflected, as a result of the reversibility of optical systems. This is brought to a focus at the far point of the eye
2. Observation of the movement of this image produced by movement of the light source allows location of this far point
3. 3 stages
   a. Illumination — using a light source reflected via a plane or concave mirror
   b. Reflex — image formation at far point
   c. Projection — location of the far point
4. Point of reversal — end point of retinoscopy after inserting trial lenses. Far point is located at examiner's sight hole
5. Observed movements using plane mirror
   a. Against — myopia of greater than working distance
   b. With — emmetropia
      — myopia of less than working distance
      — hypermetropia
6. Very accurate technique related to sight hole size
7. Errors relate to age
   a. Young, +0.5 D due to reflection at inner limiting membrane
   b. Old, −0.5 D due to reflection from deeper layers
8. Correction of astigmatism — check movement in principle meridia and correct with trial lenses using spheres or spherocylinder form

Subjective techniques

1. Pin hole test
   a. Reduces the size of the blur circle improving resolution
   b. Allows rapid differentiation between reduced vision due to ametropia and that due to pathology or amblyopia
   c. Vision not fully corrected if ametropia greater than +4.00 or −4.00 D
2. Best vision sphere (BVS) — best spherical correcting lens to provide best visual acuity. Minimum minus, maximum plus technique
3. Duochrome test
   a. Assessment of BVS

b. Utilizes ocular chromatic aberrations. Shorter wavelength, green light refracted more than red
c. Red and green targets used
d. Should be used with other methods of BVS testing
e. First impression of target clarity important
   (i) Emmetrope — equally bright targets
   (ii) Myope — red more distinct
   (iii) Hypermetrope — usually green more distinct, may accommodate to either
f. Can be used if the patient is colour blind

Jackson cross cylinder
1. Spherocylindrical lens in which the power of the sphere is half the power of the cylinder and of the opposite sign
2. Powers — + 0.25 to + 2.00 D (in 0.25 steps)
3. Uses
   a. Axis determination 1st
   b. Determination of cylinder power 2nd
4. Only of use if close to real cylinder on retinoscopy
5. Encourages active accommodation
6. Use circular targets one line above vision line on acuity chart
7. Check axis, then power and then axis again
8. 0.5 D change in cylinder requires the addition of a 0.25 D sphere of the opposite sign

Stenopaeic slit
1. Restricts blur circle in one meridian
2. Subjective technique for correction of astigmatism

Fan and block
Technique for determining the power and axis of cylinder

Appendix 1

PHOTOCOAGULATION

Relies on the absorption of light energy by ocular pigments such as xanthophyll, melanin and haemoglobin. Light energy is converted into heat. Source of light can be
1. Bright light, e.g. xenon arc lamp
2. Laser (Light Amplification by Stimulated Emission of Radiation)

Indications for photocoagulation
1. Anterior segment
   a. Eyelid tumours — removed with the carbon dioxide laser
   b. Destroying eyelash roots in trichiasis
   c. Cutting sutures
   d. Trabeculoplasty in chronic open angle glaucoma
   e. Iridotomy
   f. Pupilloplasty
   g. Photocoagulation of the ciliary processes to reduce aqueous secretion
   h. Photocoagulation of blood vessels on cornea and iris
   i. Gonioplasty
2. Posterior segment
   a. Creating adhesions around retinal holes and tears
   b. Panretinal photocoagulation for proliferative retinal disease and rubeosis
   c. Macular oedema
   d. Central serous maculopathy (improves speed of resolution but not visual prognosis)
   e. Direct photocoagulation to vascular abnormalities
   f. Intraocular tumours

Complications of photocoagulation
1. Cornea
   a. Burns
   b. Erosions
   c. Superficial punctate keratopathy or keratitis
   d. Bullous keratopathy

2. Iris
   a. Burns to iris causing iritis
   b. Iris atrophy
   c. Sphincter damage
3. Lens — lens opacities
4. Anterior chamber — shallowing of anterior chamber due to ciliochoroidal detachment. Shallowing of anterior chamber may lead to closed angle glaucoma
5. Posterior segment
   a. Foveal burn
   b. Retinal and choroidal haemorrhage
   c. Macula oedema and pucker
   d. Occlusion of vein or artery
   e. Contraction of fibrous tissue
   f. Night blindness
   g. Change in colour perception
   h. Constriction of visual fields
   i. Nerve fibre bundle defects
   j. Decrease in visual acuity

LASERS

Argon laser
1. Principle — blue-green light 488 nm and green light 515 nm. Absorbed by melanin, haemoglobin and xanthophyll. Green wavelength may be advantageous in the macular area due to reduced absorption by xanthophyll
2. Clinical uses — as above. Most frequently used ophthalmic laser

Krypton laser
1. Principle — red light 647 nm. Absorbed by melanin, but, poorly by haemoglobin and xanthophyll. Theoretical advantage over Argon
   a. Less absorbed by xanthophyll in mature lens and macula
   b. Less absorbed by vitreous haemorrhage
2. Clinical uses — predominantly retinal and macular photocoagulation

Carbon dioxide laser
1. Principle — high absorptive properties
2. Clinical uses
   a. Lid tumours
   b. Trabeculosclerostomy (hole in sclera and trabecular meshwork)
   c. Vapourizing intraocular tumours
   d. Closed end CO_2 laser probe to cauterize bleeding blood vessels or to create choroidoretinal adhesions around a tear

Neodymium Yttrium-Aluminium-Garnet (Nd-YAG) laser
1. Principle — 1064 nanometres infrared nonvisible light. Main
   use in ophthalmology is high power pulses causing optical
   breakdown and localized mechanical disruptions. This process
   does not rely on light absorption so semi-transparent
   membranes can be cut. High power pulses can be one of two
   modalities:
   a. Q(quality)-switched — usual pulse duration 10–20 ns,
      energy up to 20 mJ. Several pulses can be used in a single
      burst
   b. Mode locked — train of pulses delivered lasting ps (typically
      30 ps). Each train has 7–10 pulses with inter space pulsing
      of 5–7 ns. Whole train lasts 35–70 ns. Mode locking is now
      rarely used (The terms 'fundamental mode' and 'multi-
      mode' refer to the laser spot size)
2. Clinical uses (in Q-switched mode)
   a. Iridotomy
   b. Posterior capsulotomy
   c. Breaking of synechiae
   d. Dissection of vitreous membranes
   e. Anterior capsulotomy preoperatively
   f. Liquefaction of lens nucleus before phacoemulsification
   g. Trabeculotomy
   h. Breaking of vitreous strands (not if fluoride gas is in the eye)
   i. Cutting of intraocular lens loops
3. Complications
   a. Damage to adjoining structures in the eye including
      endothelium, trabecular meshwork, lens and retina
   b. Rise in intraocular pressure which may:
      (i) Take several weeks to develop
      (ii) Result in a pressure > 50 mmHg
      (iii) Be sustained
   The neodymium YAG laser can also be used at longer
   exposure duration and low peak power (free running). No
   optical breakdown and purely thermal interactions. Exposure
   durations 0.2–10 milliseconds
4. Clinical uses (free running)
   a. Direct treatment to the iris causing opening up of the angle
      (gonioplasty) and pupil (pupilloplasty)
   b. Closing of blood vessels on iris
   c. Trabeculoplasty
   d. Trans-scleral cyclophotocoagulation
   e. Irradiation of retina and choroid

Complications of laser iridotomy
1. Spontaneous closure
2. Uveitis
3. Corneal endothelial damage

4. Transient elevation of intraocular pressure
5. Permanent elevation of intraocular pressure
6. Hyphaema
7. Localised lens opacity
8. Pupillary distortion

Excimer lasers

1. Principle — group of lasers whose lasing activity is related to the dissociation of a molecule of an inert gas that has been forced to associate with a molecule of a halogen gas, e.g. argon fluoride excimer laser
   a. Emission wavelength 193 nm
   b. Photons from laser destabilize valency bonds of macromolecules and cause them to fall apart
   c. Photons cannot penetrate more than a few microns into tissue (hence theoretically safe for use on the cornea)
   d. Excised surface is optically smooth and sealed by a 'pseudomembrane'
2. Uses — experimental at present
   a. Fine surgical incisions in cornea
   b. By passing laser through a circular incision analogous to the trephining of a lamellar bed. A 10 D negative correction can be induced by removing only 25 μm of tissue. Major problem is healing and remoulding of cornea

Appendix 2

Visual standards for driving

(Adapted with kind permission from chapter on 'Vision' by A G Cross MD FRCS in 'Medical Aspects of Fitness to Drive' and 'Fitness to Drive' by C G Munton FRCS)

Car drivers
1. Visual acuity
   a. The standard of visual acuity which is required for drivers in the United Kingdom is the ability to read a clean car number plate with figures 3.5 inches high at twenty-five yards in bright daylight and with spectacles if worn. (The number plate figures which are 3⅛ inches high should be read at a minimum distance of 67 feet). This standard equates roughly to 6/10, although there is no direct equivalent as glare and outdoor contrast sensitivity conditions do not exist in the controlled environment of the consulting room
   b. Inability to reach this standard should be notified to the Licensing Centre by the driver
   c. EEC law for Group 1 (cars and motorcycles) requires a visual acuity of 0.4 in one eye, 0.2 in the other and 0.5 (6/12) binocularly. For one-eyed drivers the visual requirement is 0.8
2. Visual fields
   a. Persons who have only one eye can drive a car in safety.
   b. Monocular vision is not regarded as a cause for disqualification from car driving so long as the field of vision in the remaining eye is adequate (except perhaps for a short period after an eye has been removed). An adequate field is 120° on the horizontal meridian and 20° on the vertical meridian, above and below fixation measured by perimetry using a 3 mm white test object at 0.33 m (or equivalent perimetry)
   c. Unilateral amblyopia likewise does not contraindicate driving
   d. Monocular vision should be notified to the Licensing Centre

e. Binocular field defects such as bitemporal hemianopia or homonymous hemianopia, if complete or substantial in the lower quadrants, are a bar to driving

f. To drive with a field of binocular vision which is less than 120° is considered unsafe

g. EEC law for group 1 requires that no more than 20% of the temporal field may be lost

3. Diplopia

a. Paralysis of the extraocular muscles, giving rise to double vision, causes unfitness to drive

b. The use of a prismatic lens, if this overcomes diplopia, will render the patient safe to drive

c. Fluctuating degrees of diplopia and ptosis (that occur in conditions such as myasthenia gravis) are permissible if they are controlled by treatment.

d. If ocular muscular fatigue and diplopia are not controlled by treatment, driving should not be allowed

e. Patients should not be allowed to drive if they are subject to transient attacks of diplopia

f. Patients with diplopia should notify the Licensing Centre of their disability

4. Colour vision

a. Patients with defective colour vision may drive.

b. Investigation has failed to show any significant correlation between defective colour vision and road accidents

5. Dark adaptation

a. The more marked degrees of night vision defect occur in diseases such as retinitis pigmentosa and advanced choroidoretinitis

b. These conditions should be regarded as obstacles to driving, and should be notified to the Licensing Centre

Drivers of heavy goods and public service vehicles, and other professional drivers. EEC Group 2 (vehicles exceeding 3500 kg or exceeding 8 passengers plus driver, or a combination of these)
The current recommendations which have been implemented by the Traffic Commissioners are as follows:

1. Visual Acuity

a. The uncorrected static visual acuity must be at least 6/60 (soon to be amended to 3/60) in each eye, and the corrected vision must be at least 6/9 in one eye and 6/12 in the other

b. Provided a vocational driver complies with the minimum requirements for static visual acuity, there should be no bar to the wearing of contact lenses

c. Persons who held an HGV or PSV licence prior to 1 January 1983 may continue to hold a vocational driving licence providing they can meet a corrected standard of visual acuity of 6/12 in the better eye and 6/36 in the worse eye

2. Pathological field defects
   Any pathological visual field defect should be a bar to the
   holding of a licence to drive a HGV or PSV
3. Diplopia
   Insuperable diplopia should be a bar to the holding of a licence
   to drive a HGV or PSV
4. Monocularism
   a. Monocularism should not be acceptable in new applicants
      for HGV and PSV licences
   b. Existing licence holders who become monocular should be
      required to surrender their HGV and PSV licences
   c. The renewal of licences for drivers who are already
      monocular should be a matter for the licencing authority to
      determine according to the circumstances of the particular
      case, and with appropriate medical advice
5. Cataract operations
   a. A driver who has had a cataract operation with an
      intraocular implant may be allowed to drive a HGV or PSV
      two months after the operation if he fulfills the necessary
      visual standards
   b. However, visual acuity should be checked every year
6. Impaired colour vision
   This should not be an impediment to the holding of a HGV or
   PSV licence
7. Night-time visual standards
   Special night-time visual standards are not considered at
   present

Table 11 Approximate equivalents for common perimeters on a theoretical basis

	Perimeter	Goldman	Cooper-Dicon	Humphrey	Octopus	Fieldmaster
Target size	3/330 white	Target III = 4 mm Filters 4e	—		—	—
Angle	0.52°	0.7°	<0.5°	<0.5°	<0.5°	—
Bowl luminance	<3 Asb	31.5 Asb	31.5 Asb	31.5 Asb	4 Asb	31.5 Asb
Target luminance	38–75 Asb	1000 Asb	315–3150 Asb	3150 Asb	Dependent on strategy & algorithm	—
Target brightness over background	15 dB	15 dB	10–20 dB	20 dB	(20 dB)	10–20 dB

Appendix 3

(Reproduced in part from the BD8 form by kind permission of the Department of Health and Social Security)

Definition of blindness

1. The statutory definition for the purposes of registration as a blind person under the National Assistance Act 1948, is that the person is 'so blind as to be unable to perform any work for which eyesight is essential'

Note
   a. The test is not whether the person is unable to pursue his ordinary occupation or any other ocupation, but whether he is too blind to perform *any work* for which eyesight is essential.
   b. Only the visual conditions are taken into account and other bodily or mental infirmities are disregarded
2. The principal condition to be considered is the visual acuity (i.e. the best direct vision available with each eye or both together, where both are present, as tested by Snellen's type with focus properly corrected), but regard must also be paid to the other conditions set out below.
3. The persons examined may be classified in three groups as follows:
Group 1 — $< 3/60$ Snellen
In general, a person with visual acuity below $3/60$ may be regarded as blind.
Group 2 — $3/60-<6/60$ Snellen
A person with visual acuity of at least $3/60$ but less than $6/60$ Snellen
   a. may be regarded as blind if the field of vision is considerably contracted, but
   b. should not be regarded as blind if the visual defect is of long standing and is unaccompanied by any material contraction of the field of vision, e.g. in cases of congenital nystagmus, albinism, myopia etc.
Group 3 — $\geqslant 6/60$ Snellen
A person with a visual acuity of $6/60$ or better should not normally be regarded as blind. He may, however, be regarded

as blind if the field of vision is markedly contracted in the greater part of its extent, and particularly if the contraction is in the lower part of the field; but a person suffering from homonymous or bitemporal hemianopia retaining central visual acuity of 6/18 or better is not to be regarded as blind

Notes

a. The question of whether a defect of vision is recent or of long standing has a special bearing on the certification of blindness. A person whose defect is recent is less able to adapt himself to his environment than is a person with the same visual acuity whose defect has been of long standing. This is specially applicable to Groups 2 and 3

b. Another factor of importance, particularly in relation to Group 2, is the age of the person at the onset of blindness. An old person with a recent failure of sight cannot adapt himself as readily as a younger person with the same defect

c. On rare occasions cases will arise which are not precisely covered by the foregoing observations, and such cases must be dealt with according to the judgement of the certifying ophthalmic surgeon

d. In making recommendations about persons up to and including the age of sixteen, examining ophthalmologists should bear in mind that there are other factors which may influence local education authorities in their decision about the special educational treatment to be provided

Definition of partial sight

1. There is no statutory definition in the National Assistance Act 1948 for partial sight, but the Ministry of Health has advised that the person who is not blind within the meaning of the 1948 Act, but who is nevertheless substantially and permanently handicapped by congenitally defective vision, or in whose case illness or injury has caused defective vision of a substantial or permanently handicapping character is within the scope of the welfare services which the local authority are empowered to provide for blind persons; but this does not apply to other benefits specially enjoyed by the blind, e.g. income tax concession where eligible

2. The following criteria should be used as a general guide when determining whether a person falls within the scope of the welfare provisions for the partially sighted, as well as in recommending, where the person is under the age of sixteen years, the appropriate type of school for the particular child concerned:

  a. for registration purposes and the provision of welfare
     services, those with visual acuity
     (i) 3/60 to 6/60 with full field
     (ii) up to 6/24 with moderate contraction of the field,
          opacities in media, or aphakia
     (iii) 6/18 or even better if there is a gross field defect, e.g.
           hemianopia, or there is a marked contraction of the field
           as in pigmentary degeneration, glaucoma etc
  b. for children whose visual acuity will have a bearing on the
     appropriate methods of education
     (i) severe visual disabilities — to be educated in special
         schools by methods involving vision — 3/60 to 6/24
         with glasses
     (ii) visual impairment — to be educated at ordinary schools
          by special consideration — better than 6/24 with
          glasses

Notes
  a. Infants and young children with congenital anomalies,
     including visual defects, unless obviously blind should be
     classed as being partially sighted
  b. At age four and over, binocular corrected vision should be
     the criterion
  c. All in 2b (i) and (ii) above should be re-examined every 12
     months, or earlier if there is reason to suspect any
     deterioration
  d. In making recommendations about persons up to and
     including the age of sixteen, examining ophthalmologists
     should bear in mind that — as with blindness — there are
     other factors which may influence local education
     authorities in their decision about the special education
     treatment to be provided

FURTHER READING

Clinical ophthalmology

Chignell A H 1980 *Retinal Detachment Surgery* Springer-Verlag, Berlin (ISBN 3-540-09475)

Dorrell E D 1978 *Surgery of the Eye* Blackwell, Oxford (ISBN 0-632-00122-4)

Duane T D 1986 *Clinical Ophthalmology* Harper and Row, Philadelphia (ISBN 0-06-148007-X)

Gittinger Jr J W, Asdourian G K 1988 *Manual of Clinical Problems in Ophthalmology* Little Brown, Boston (ISBN 0-316-31472-2)

Kanski J J 1984 *Clinical Ophthalmology* Butterworths, London (ISBN 0-407-00295-2)

Kanski J J 1985 *Retinal Detachment* Butterworths, London (ISBN 0-407-00421-1)

Mein J, Harcourt B 1986 *Diagnosis and Management of Ocular Motility Disorders* Blackwell, Oxford (ISBN 0-632-01589-6)

Miller S J (ed) 1987 *Clinical Ophthalmology* John Wright, Bristol (ISBN 0-7236-0754-0)

Newell F W 1982 *Ophthalmology* C V Mosby, St Louis (ISBN 000010336)

Spalton D J, Hitchings R A, Hunter P A 1984 *Atlas of Clinical Ophthalmology* Churchill Livingstone, Edinburgh (ISBN 0-443-03115-0)

Trevor-Roper P D, Curran P V 1984 *The Eye and its Disorders* Blackwell, Oxford (ISBN 0-632-01003-7)

Optics and refraction

Duke-Elder S 1978 *The Practice of Refraction* Churchill Livingstone, Edinburgh (ISBN 0-443-01478-7)

Elkington A R, Frank H 1984 *Clinical Optics* Blackwell, Oxford (ISBN 0-632-01149-1)

Neurology and general medicine

Ashworth B 1973 *Clinical Neuro-ophthalmology* Blackwell, Oxford, (ISBN 0-632-07960-6)

Clifford-Rose F (ed) 1983 *The Eye in General Medicine* Chapman and Hall, London (ISBN 0-412-24760-7)

Dinning W J 1987 *Systemic inflammatory Disease and the Eye* John Wright, Bristol (ISBN 0-7236-0777 X)

Kanski J J 1985 *The Eye in Systemic Disease* Butterworths, London (ISBN 0-407-00417-3)

Pattern J 1977 *Neurological Differential Diagnosis* Harold Starke, London (ISBN 0-287-66988-2)

Rubenstein D, Wayne D 1980 *Lecture Notes in Clinical Medicine* Blackwell, Oxford (ISBN 0-632-00545-9)

Basic sciences and pathology

Adler F H 1987 *Physiology of the Eye* C V Mosby, St Louis (ISBN LC86-016180)

Davson H 1980 *Physiology of the Eye* Churchill Livingstone, Edinburgh (ISBN 0-443-01892-8)

Greer C H 1979 *Ocular pathology* Blackwell, Oxford (ISBN 0-632-00469-X)

Wolff E 1976 *Anatomy of the Eye and Orbit* H K Lewis, London (ISBN 0-7186-0426-1)

Journals

American Journal of Ophthalmology
Archives of Ophthalmology
British Journal of Ophthalmology
British Medical Journal
Eye (Transactions of the Ophthalmological Society of the United Kingdom)
Survey of Ophthalmology

Index